Lecture Notes in Computer Science 10555

Commenced Publication in 1973
Founding and Former Series Editors:
Gerhard Goos, Juris Hartmanis, and Jan van Leeuwen

More information about this series at http://www.springer.com/series/7412

M. Jorge Cardoso · Tal Arbel et al. (Eds.)

Molecular Imaging, Reconstruction and Analysis of Moving Body Organs, and Stroke Imaging and Treatment

Fifth International Workshop, CMMI 2017
Second International Workshop, RAMBO 2017
and First International Workshop, SWITCH 2017
Held in Conjunction with MICCAI 2017
Québec City, QC, Canada, September 14, 2017
Proceedings

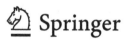 Springer

Editors
M. Jorge Cardoso
University College London
London
UK

Tal Arbel
McGill University
Montreal, QC
Canada

Workshop Editors *see next page*

ISSN 0302-9743 ISSN 1611-3349 (electronic)
Lecture Notes in Computer Science
ISBN 978-3-319-67563-3 ISBN 978-3-319-67564-0 (eBook)
DOI 10.1007/978-3-319-67564-0

Library of Congress Control Number: 2017953410

LNCS Sublibrary: SL6 – Image Processing, Computer Vision, Pattern Recognition, and Graphics

Printed on acid-free paper

This Springer imprint is published by Springer Nature
The registered company is Springer International Publishing AG
The registered company address is: Gewerbestrasse 11, 6330 Cham, Switzerland

Workshop Editors

Fifth International Workshop on Computational Methods for Molecular Imaging, CMMI 2017

Fei Gao
Siemens Medical Solutions
Knoxville, TN
USA

Kuangyu Shi
Technical University of Munich
Munich
Germany

Second International Workshop on Reconstruction and Analysis of Moving Body Organs, RAMBO 2017

Bernhard Kainz
Imperial College London
London
UK

Tom Vercauteren
University College London
London
UK

Kanwal K. Bhatia
Visulytix Limited
London
UK

First International Stroke Workshop on Imaging and Treatment Challenges, SWITCH 2017

Theo van Walsum
Erasmus MC
Rotterdam
The Netherlands

Mauricio Reyes
University of Bern
Bern
Switzerland

Roman Peter
Erasmus MC
Rotterdam
The Netherlands

Roland Wiest
University Hospital of Bern
Bern
Switzerland

Wiro Niessen
Erasmus MC
Rotterdam
The Netherlands

Bart J. Emmer
Academic Medical Center
Amsterdam
The Netherlands

Adrian Dalca
Harvard Medical School
Boston, MA
USA

Preface CMMI 2017

Molecular imaging is an evolving clinical and research discipline enabling the visualization, characterization, and quantification of biological processes taking place at the cellular and subcellular levels within intact living subjects. As a dedicated workshop, Computational Methods for Molecular Imaging (CMMI 2017) covered various areas from image synthesis to data analysis and from clinical diagnosis to therapy individualization, using molecular imaging modalities PET, SPECT, PET/CT, SPECT/CT, and PET/MR. Technical topics included image reconstruction, image enhancement, physiological modeling, computational simulation, multi-modal analysis, and artificial intelligence methods with clear clinical application and close industrial connection.

September 2017

Fei Gao
Kuangyu Shi

Organization

Organizing Committee

Fei Gao	Siemens Medical Solutions, USA
Kuangyu Shi	Technical University of Munich, Germany

Steering Committee

Nassir Navab	Technical University of Munich, Germany
Sibylle Ziegler	University of Munich, Germany
Pengcheng Shi	Rochester Institute of Technology, USA
Julia Schnabel	King's College London, UK

Program Committee

Ulas Bagci	University of Central Florida, USA
Michael Brady	Oxford University, UK
Ralph Buchert	Charité Berlin, Germany
Cyrill Burger	PMOD, Switzerland
Weidong Cai	University of Sydney, Australia
David Dagan Feng	University of Sydney, Australia
Roger Gunn	Imperial College London, UK
Sung-Cheng (Henry) Huang	University of California at Los Angeles, USA
Hidehiro Lida	National Institute of Radiology Sciences, Japan
Jieqing Jiao	University College London, UK
Jinman Kim	University of Sydney and Nepean Hospital, Australia
Adriaan Lammertsma	VU University Medical Center, The Netherlands
Huafeng Liu	Zhejiang University, China
Su Ruan	University of Rouen, France
Jie Tian	CAS, China
Harry Tsoumpas	University of Leeds, UK
Luping Zhou	University of Wollongang, Australia
Yun Zhou	Johns Hopkins University, USA
Hongli Li	United Imaging, USA

Preface RAMBO 2017

Physiological motion is an important factor in several medical imaging applications. The speed of motion may inhibit the acquisition of high-resolution images needed for effective visualisation and analysis, for example in cardiac or respiratory imaging or in fMRI and perfusion applications. Additionally, in cardiac and fetal imaging, the variation in frame of reference may confound automated analysis pipelines. The underlying motion may also need to be characterised either to enhance images or for clinical assessment. Techniques are therefore needed for faster or more accurate reconstruction or for analysis of time-dependent images. Despite the related concerns, few meetings have focused on the issues caused by motion in medical imaging, without restriction on the clinical application area or methodology used.

After a very successful international workshop on Reconstruction and Analysis of Moving Body Organs (RAMBO) at MICCAI 2016 in Athens, Greece, we are proud to have organised this meeting for the second time in conjunction with MICCAI 2017 in Quebec, Canada.

RAMBO was set up to provide a discussion forum for researchers for whom motion and its effects on image analysis or visualisation is a key aspect of their work. By inviting contributions across all application areas, the workshop aimed to bring together ideas from different areas of specialisation, without being confined to a particular methodology. In particular, the recent trend to move from model-based to learning-based methods of analysis has resulted in increased transferability between application domains. A further goal of this workshop series is to enhance the links between image analysis (including computer vision and machine learning techniques) and image acquisition and reconstruction, which generally tends to be addressed in separate meetings.

The presented contributions can be broadly categorised into "registration and tracking" and "image reconstruction and information retrieval", while application areas include cardiac, pulmonal, abdominal, fetal, and renal imaging, showing the breadth of interest in the topic. Research from both academia and industry is presented and keynote lectures from Dr. Aleksandra Popovic (Philips Research North America) and Prof. Ali Gholipour (Harvard Medical School) give an overview of recent developments.

We believe that this workshop fosters the cross-fertilisation of ideas across application domains while tackling and taking advantage of the problems and opportunities arising from motion in medical imaging.

September 2017

Bernhard Kainz
Kanwal Bhatia
Tom Vercauteren

Organization

Organizing Committee

Bernhard Kainz	Imperial College London, UK
Kanwal Bhatia	King's College London and Visulytix, UK
Tom Vercauteren	University College London, UK

Program Committee

Wenjia Bai	Imperial College London, UK
Aurelien Bustin	King's College London, UK
Lucilio Cordero-Grande	King's College London, UK
Nishikant Deshmukh	Johns Hopkins University, USA
Ali Gholipour	Boston Children's Hospital, USA
Alberto Gomez	King's College London, UK
Matthias Heinrich	Universität zu Lübeck, Germany
Yipeng Hu	University College London, UK
Karim Lekadir	Stanford University, USA
Roxane Licandro	Vienna University of Technology, Austria
Herve Lombaert	ETS Montreal, Canada
Keelin Murphy	University College Cork, Ireland
Ozan Oktay	Imperial College London, UK
Bishesh Khanal	King's College London UK
Bartlomiej Papiez	University of Oxford, UK
Francois Rousseau	Télécom Bretagne, France
Martin Urschler	Graz University of Technology, Austria
Wolfgang Wein	ImFusion GmbH, Germany

Preface SWITCH 2017

The first Stroke Workshop on Imaging and Treatment Challenges (SWITCH) was held at the Medical Image Computing and Computer Assisted Intervention Conference (MICCAI) in Quebec City, Canada, 2017.

The SWITCH workshop focused on the challenges in the management of stroke patients, particularly regarding diagnostic imaging and treatment. The purpose of this workshop was to introduce the clinical background of challenges/opportunities related to imaging for stroke to the imaging community and to stimulate discussion and the exchange of ideas. The SWITCH half-day workshop joined the MICCAI initiative for bundled joint proceedings of the satellite events together with the Ischemic Stroke Lesion Segmentation (ISLES) Challenge.

The SWITCH workshop organizing committee consisted of scientists and clinical experts from the Erasmus MC, Delft University of Technology, Massachusetts Institute of Technology, Harvard Medical School, the University of Bern, the University Hospital of Bern, and Amsterdam Medical Center.

The challenges in stroke imaging were addressed by three clinical keynote speakers, Dr. Roland Wiest (University Hospital of Bern) on MR imaging, and Dr. Kambiz Nael (Icahn School of Medicine at Mount Sinai) on CT imaging and Dr. Vitor Mendes Pereira (Toronto Western Hospital) on stroke interventions.

The papers submitted for this workshop were evaluated by two independent scientific reviewers each, whose affiliations were checked to avoid conflict of interest, and all four papers were included in the proceedings. The topics addressed in these papers focus on CT(A)-based quantitative imaging biomarkers for stroke.

The organizers of the two workshops would like to express their sincere thanks to the keynote speakers, the authors of the contributed papers, and the attendees of the workshops. A special word of thanks goes to the sponsors, Olea Medical and Philips Healthcare, who facilitated the contributions of the clinical keynote speakers at the workshop.

September 2017

Theo van Walsum
Roman Peter
Wiro Niessen
Adrian Dalca
Mauricio Reyes
Roland Wiest
Bart Emmer

Organization

Organizing Committee

Theo van Walsum	Erasmus MC, The Netherlands
Roman Peter	Erasmus MC, The Netherlands
Wiro Niessen	Erasmus MC, and Delft University of Technology, The Netherlands
Adrian Dalca	Harvard Medical School, USA
Mauricio Reyes	University of Bern, Switzerland
Roland Wiest	Inselspital Bern, Switzerland
Bart Emmer	Amsterdam Medical Center, The Netherlands

Program Committee

Theo van Walsum	Erasmus MC, The Netherlands
Roman Peter	Erasmus MC, The Netherlands
Wiro Niessen	Erasmus MC, and Delft University of Technology, The Netherlands
Adrian Dalca	Harvard Medical School, USA
Mauricio Reyes	University of Bern, Switzerland
Roland Wiest	Inselspital Bern, Switzerland
Bart Emmer	Amsterdam Medical Center, The Netherlands

Contents

**First International Stroke Workshop on Imaging
and Treatment Challenges, SWITCH 2017**

Fifth International Workshop on Computational Methods for Molecular Imaging, CMMI 2017

3D Lymphoma Segmentation in PET/CT Images Based on Fully Connected CRFs

Yuntao Yu[1,2], Pierre Decazes[2], Isabelle Gardin[2], Pierre Vera[2], and Su Ruan[1(✉)]

[1] Université de Rouen, LITIS EA 4108, 76031 Rouen, France
yu.yuntao@hotmail.com, su.ruan@univ-rouen.fr
[2] CHB Hospital, Rue d'Amiens, CS11516 76038 Rouen Cedex1, France
{pierre.decazes, isabelle.gardin,
pierre.vera}@chb.unicancer.fr

Abstract. Positron Emission Tomography (PET) is widely used for lymphoma detection. It is often combined with the CT scan in order to provide anatomical information for helping lymphoma detection. Two common types of approaches can be distinguished for lymphoma detection and segmentation in PET. The first one is ROI dependent which needs a ROI defined by physicians who firstly detect where lymphomas are. The second one is based on machine learning methods which need a large learning database. However, such a large standard database is quite rare in medical field. Considering these problems, we propose a new approach which combines a multi-atlas segmentation of the CT with CRFs (Conditional Random Fields) segmentation method in PET. It consists of 3 steps. Firstly, an anatomical multi-atlas segmentation is applied on CT to locate and remove the organs having hyper metabolism in PET. Secondly, CRFs detect and segment the lymphoma regions in PET. The conditional probabilities used in CRFs are usually estimated by a learning step. In this work, we propose to estimate them in an unsupervised way. A list of the detected regions in 3D is visualized. The final step is to select real lymphomas by simply clicking on them. Our method is tested on ten patients. The rate of good detection is 100%. The average of Dice index over 10 patients for measuring the lymphoma is 80% compared to manual lymphoma segmentation. Comparing with other methods in terms of Dice index shows the best performance of our method.

Keywords: Positron Emission Tomography (PET) · Lymphoma segmentation · Fully connected conditional random fields · Anatomical atlas

1 Introduction

Positron Emission Tomography (PET) is a nuclear medicine functional imaging technique which can observe the metabolic activity of tumors. Despite of the low resolution and poor SNR as described in [1], the positron emission tomography using 18F-FDG is still one of the most widely used approaches for the lymphoma detection, as most lymphoma subtypes have high (18)F-FDG avidity [17].

Lymphoma is a group of blood cancers which develops in lymphatic system. Its high morbidity and mortality has drawn an important attention by doctors and related

© Springer International Publishing AG 2017
M.J. Cardoso et al. (Eds.): CMMI/RAMBO/SWITCH 2017, LNCS 10555, pp. 3–12, 2017.
DOI: 10.1007/978-3-319-67564-0_1

researchers. In particular, it has been shown that the whole volume of the lymphoma is an important prognostic factor [18] which supports the need to find an algorithm measuring automatically the volume of the disease. To identify a lymphoma from PET/CT scan needs to overcome the following difficulties. Firstly, lymphoma's metabolism on PET image in terms of standardized uptake value (SUV) [15] is not fixed. Its metabolism varies from different patients, subtypes of lymphoma and severities. Secondly, as lymphatic system belongs circulatory system, lymphoma can appear in many parts of body. In addition, the form of lymphoma varies from one to another and it contains very little texture information, as shown in Fig. 1.

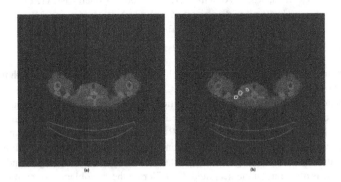

Fig. 1. (a) Combination of PET image (in red) and CT scan. (b) The ground truth of lymphoma sites contoured in yellow in PET and CT. (Color figure online)

The lack of image characteristic information of lymphoma makes it difficult to be automatically detected. Different approaches have been reported for this task in the literature. They can be separated into two common types. The first type consists of ROI-dependent methods, where the ROI is usually defined by a doctor with a human time-consuming processing. The most widely used segmentation approach of this type in clinical application is thresholding by 40% of the maximum SUV in ROI. But in several particular situations, when SUV values in the ROI are not homogeneous, this threshold approach using fixed-value can provide a poor result. Thus, different methods [8, 9, 10] are proposed to improve it. Vauclin's method [10] uses a no linear model to find the threshold by an iterative way. Cellule automata (CA) [2] is based on region growing approach with seeds distributed in a ROI. Second type of lymphoma detection and segmentation approach does not need a ROI a priori, it uses machine learning by learning and analyzing a huge database. Different features of lymphoma are learnt and trained from PET image. The main methods of this second type of approach are SVM [12], Random Forest and Component-Trees [3], recently deep learning [13].

As the lymphoma can appear in many parts in the body and the number of lymphoma can be important, definition of ROI increases largely doctors' work. In addition, the results of segmentation are highly related with the defined ROI. The second type of approach is promising. However, it needs a standard and global admitted database which is hard to get. So, our approach tries to use another way to segment the lymphoma. It combines an anatomical atlas obtained in CT and a fully connected conditional random fields based segmentation to detect and segment automatically lymphoma regions in 3D. Firstly, the anatomical multi-atlas segmentation of the CT removes the organs on the PET which have a physiological hyper metabolism and which are usually not affected by the disease: brain, heart, kidneys and bladder. We use the method proposed in [14] for this step. After removing these organs, the CRFs algorithm is applied on the PET image volume for lymphoma detection and segmentation. The CRFs model is composed by a unary energy and Gaussian kernel pairwise energy. The conditional probabilities used in the unary energy are usually estimated by a learning step. In this work, we propose to estimate the probability of lymphoma in an unsupervised way. It combines k-means clustering algorithm and a model based on sigmoid function. The pairwise energy includes the contrast and the spatial distance information in order to improve segmentation results. And finally, all the detected regions are visualized in 3D, allowing the user to select the lymphoma to be studied by simply clicking on it. This interaction allows to largely reduce the time comparing to the creation of ROI on whole patient body.

In this paper, we focus on the development of CRFs based segmentation. The paper's structure is as follows: Sect. 2 presents our CRFs model and related inference; Sect. 3 explains our evaluation metrics, the parameters' estimation and our obtained results comparing to other segmentation algorithms; Conclusion and perspectives are given in the last section.

2   Method

CRFs algorithm is applied widely in natural language processing and sequential data labelling or parsing. Recent researches show also its significant application in object recognition and multi-class image segmentation [4, 5]. To our knowledge, our work is the first application of the fully connected CRFs on PET image.

2.1   The Fully Connected CRFs Model

Consider $C = \{c_1, c_2, ..., c_l\}$ is a set of class with l representing the number of class. The conditional probability of the class C on image $X = \{x_1, x_2, ..., x_N\}$, where N is the number of pixels and x_i SUV value of the voxel i, is defined as:

$$log\, P(C|X, \theta) = \sum\nolimits_i U(C_i, x_i; \theta_u) + \sum\nolimits_{i,j} V\left(C_i, C_j, x_i, x_j; \theta_v\right) - log\, Z(\theta, X) \quad (1)$$

where U is the unary potential on each voxel and V is the pairwise potential between two voxels i and j, $Z(\theta, X)$ the partition function which normalizes the distribution, C_i the related label for voxel i. $\theta = \{\theta_u, \theta_v\}$ contains the unary potential parameters θ_u and the pairwise potential parameters θ_v. The unary potential proposed in the literature is usually estimated by a supervised learning step, such as DCNN (Deep convolutional neural networks) in [5]. We propose in this work a mathematical model using medical knowledge in CT and PET and a clustering algorithm.

In our case $C = \{c_{lymphoma}, c_{background}\}$ and X is SUV values in PET. To define the unary potential, we first group all voxels into k clusters. The SUV distribution of each cluster can be considered as a Gaussian distribution. Then we use Gaussian Mixture Models (GMMs) [4] where the mixture coefficients depend on the class label C to define the unary potential which is described as follow:

$$U(C_i, x_i; \theta_u) = log \sum_k p(C_i/k)P(k|x_i) \tag{2}$$

where k is cluster number. The total number of clusters is fixed by user. In our experiment, we choose 10 clusters. k-means algorithm is applied to obtain the k clusters. $p(X \mid k)$ is considered as Gaussian distribution and can be calculated from:

$$p(X|k) \sim N(X|\mu_k, \sigma_k) \tag{3}$$

As $P(x_i|k) \propto P(k|x_i)$ according to Bayes rule [4]. $P(k|x_i)$ can then be calculated by (3). To find $p(C_i|k)$, we propose a sigmoid function as follow (details in Sect. 3.3):

$$p(C_{lymphome}|k) = \textbf{Sigmoid}(\mu_k, a, b) = \frac{1}{1 + e^{-a(\mu_k - b)}} p(C_{background}|k)$$
$$= 1 - \textbf{Sigmoid}(\mu_k, a, b) = \frac{1}{1 + e^{-a(\mu_k - b)}} \tag{4}$$

where $a(a = 0.05$ in our experiments) determines the degree of the sigmoid slope, μ_k is the average of the k th cluster, b is the translation value along horizontal axis to be determined by a prior knowledge.

Concerning the pairwise potential, we use the same model as described in [5]:

$$\sum_{i,j} V(C_i, C_j, x_i, x_j; w, \theta_v) =$$

$$-\sum_{i,j} Potts(C_i, C_j) \left[exp\left(-\frac{|y_i - y_j|^2}{2\theta_\alpha^2} - \frac{|x_i - x_j|^2}{2\theta_\beta^2} \right) + w\, exp\left(-\frac{|y_i - y_j|^2}{2\theta_\Upsilon^2} \right) \right] \tag{5}$$

where $w, \theta_v = \{\theta_\alpha, \theta_\beta, \theta_\Upsilon\}$ are the parameters to be estimated, y_i and y_j coordinates of voxels i and j, $Potts(C_i, C_j)$=1 if $C_i \neq C_j$, otherwise =0. A Potts model is used to spatial labelling regularization. The objective of appearance kernel is to encourage the nearby pixels with similar SUV values to have the same label. θ_α and θ_β decide how important the spatial nearness and intensity similarity are. The smoothness kernel with θ_Υ considers only the impact of the nearest neighborhood. This pairwise potential allows to remove small isolated regions [4].

2.2 Inference of CRFs Model

The final label C^f for X is obtained by maximizing $\log P(C|X, \theta)$. As $\log Z(\theta, X)$ is the normalization term in (1), the energy to be maximized becomes:

$$J = \sum_i U(C_i, x_i; \theta_u) + \sum_{i,j} V(C_i, C_j, x_i, x_j; \theta_v) \qquad (6.1)$$

We can also minimize –J to obtain C^f:

$$C^f = \underset{c}{argmin} - \left[\sum_i U(C_i, x_i; \theta_u) + \sum_{i,j} V(C_i, C_j, x_i, x_j; \theta_v) \right] \qquad (6.2)$$

Many algorithms can be used for this energy minimization problem, such as ICM [16], alpha-expansion graph-cut [6, 11], mean field approximation [5, 7] etc. In our case, there are only two classes, so a simple ICM algorithm is used. ICM can give a local optimal solution. However, if we have a good initialization of C, we can find the global optimal solution and also reduce the converging time.

3 Evaluation and Results

3.1 Database

PET images were acquired by a PET/CT scanner (Biograph Sensation 16; Siemens, Knoxville, TN), which includes a 16-slice CT component and a PET system with lutetium oxyorthosilicate crystals. For PET imaging, the emission data were acquired from the base of the skull to the proximal thigh with acquisitions of 3 to 3.5 min per bed position, depending on the patient's body mass index (BMI), each covering 16.2 cm, at an axial sampling thickness of 2 mm per slice. The CT scan parameters were set to 100–120 kVp and 100–150 mAs (based on the patient's BMI) using dose reduction software (CareDose; Siemens Medical Solutions, Knoxville, TN). Both the PET scans and the CT scans were obtained during normal tidal breathing. The PET images were reconstructed with attenuation correction using the CT-derived data and an attenuation-weighted ordered-subsets expectation maximization (AW-OSEM) algorithm. The spatial resolution was 5.3 mm × 5.3 mm × 2 mm.

Each patient has approximately two tumor sites of Hodgkin's lymphoma. Among 10 studied patients, we have 21 tumor sites to analyze with their manual references. The average volume of lymphomas is 100.77 cm3 corresponding to 1800 voxels.

3.2 Evaluation Metrics

We separate two kinds of evaluation metrics: region based one is for detection performance, while voxel based is for segmentation. The labelled voxels with lymphoma after CRF are grouped into 3D regions by 26 convexities. One 3D region presents one lymphoma.

Considering that A is a set of ground truth regions, $\mathbf{G} = \{G_1, G_2,..., G_{ng}\}$. Each region G_i is composed of g_i voxels. B is a set of the segmented lymphoma regions,

$\mathbf{B} = \{B_1, B_2,..., B_{np}\}$. Each region B_i is composed of b_i voxels. And for each region in $\mathbf{B}$, we have $\cup_{j=1,...,ng} (B_i \cap G_j) \neq \emptyset$. $\mathbf{S}$ is a set of detected false regions, $\mathbf{S} = \{S_1, S_2,...,$ $S_{nn}\}$. Each region S_i is composed of s_i voxels. And for each region in $\mathbf{S}$, we have $\cup_{j=1,...,ng} (S_i \cap G_j) = \emptyset$. F(M) defines the number of elements in set M.

The first metric is Dice index defined for evaluating the segmented lymphoma regions:

$$DICE_{ref} = \frac{2 * F(G \cap B)}{F(G) + F(B)}$$

The second metric is different from the first DICE index by adding S:

$$DICE_{global} = \frac{2 * F[B \cap G]}{F(G) + F(B) + F(S)}$$

$DICE_{global}$ indicates the accuracy of the segmentation in a global way. This metric can have some problems if the false positive regions are important. Thus, it's wise to calculate $DICE_{ref}$ and $DICE_{global}$ separately for assessment.

For evaluating the false positive region volume, the third metric is defined by:

$$VOLUME_{sup} = \frac{F(S)}{F(B \cup S)}$$

The fourth metric is rate of true positive detected region (*Sensitivity*) indicates the rate of the truth lymphoma detected regions to all detected ones. If sensitivity equals to 1, it means all the ground truth lymphomas have been detected.

3.3   Estimation of the Parameters in CRF Model

As mentioned in Sect. 3, $P(C_i|k)$ is modeled by a sigmoid function (4), shown in Fig. 2. We propose to determinate the parameter according to the medical knowledge.

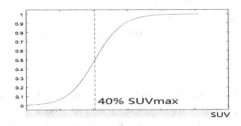

Fig. 2. Illustration of the sigmoid function. 40% SUVmax value corresponds to the parameter b in (4).

In clinical application [19], 40% SUV_{max} of local ROI thresholding is widely used for lymphoma detection and volume measurement. The result of 40% SUV_{max} thresholding is close to the manual reference. Thus b is chosen to equal to 40% estimated SUV_{max}, which means if $\mu_k^i > 40\%$ of the estimated SUVmax, the voxel i in cluster k has more than 50% chance to belong to the lymphoma. The estimated SUV_{max} can supported by Deauville five-point scale [20], which is recommended for response assessment in international guidelines and which have been validated in most lymphoma subtypes [21]. The following table shows the definition of Deauville five-point scale (Table 1).

Table 1. Definition of Deauville five-point scale [21]. The scale sores the most intense uptake in a site if initial disease, if present.

Deauville score	Definition
1	No uptake
2	Uptake $\leq$ mediastinum
3	Uptake > mediastinal but $\leq$ liver
4	Moderately increased uptake compare to the liver
5	Markedly increased uptake compared to the liver and/or new lesions
X	New areas of uptake unlikely to be related to lymphoma

Deauville Score 1 to 3, i.e. a metabolism of the target below the normal hepatic metabolism, is in favor of a PET-negative exam with an inactive disease and Deauville Score 4 and 5, i.e. a metabolism of the target above the normal hepatic metabolism, is if favor of a PET-positive exam with an active disease. The liver metabolism can therefore be used as a reference metabolism to detect the pathological metabolism [21]. Thus, we can estimate SUV_{max} as d* SUV_{liver}, where d (≥ 2.5) is a user selected float. In addition, the SUV_{liver} can be calculated in the liver region defined by an anatomical multi-atlas segmentation the CT. In our experience, d = 3.

To estimate the pairwise potential parameters: w and $\theta_v = \{\theta_\alpha, \theta_\beta, \theta_\gamma\}$, a grid search method is used as described in [5]. Since the results are not very sensible to the smoothness kernel, we fix $w = 1$ and $\theta_\gamma = 0.8$. We study the impact of the parameters $\{\theta_\alpha, \theta_\beta\}$ to the final result. The Fig. 3 shows how $\theta_\alpha, \theta_\beta$ influence the segmentation results by measuring $DICE_{ref}$, $DICE_{global}$, $VOLUME_{sup}$, Sensitivity.

By changing θ_α (theta1) and θ_β (theta2) from 3 to 30, the results of $DICE_{ref}$, $DICE_{global}$, $VOLUME_{sup} = 1$, and SENSITIVITY show that when $\theta_\alpha = 15$, $\theta_\beta = 10$, the best results are obtained: $DICE_{ref} = 82.8\%$, $DICE_{global} = 77.6\%$, $VOLUME_{sup} = 11.6\%$, SENSITIVITY = 100%. We can see also that θ_α is not sensible to the result.

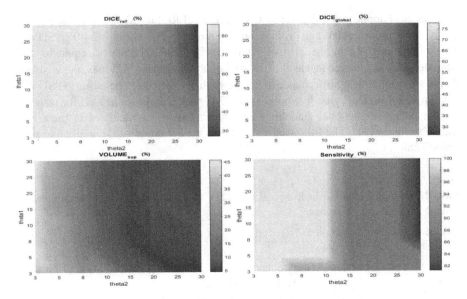

Fig. 3. Impact of the parameters $\theta_\alpha(theta1)$ and $\theta_\beta(theta2)$ to the four evaluation metrics.

3.4 Results

Our method with the estimated parameters is applied on ten patients. We compare our results with different ROI dependent methods in [2] by calculating $DICE_{ref}$, shown in Table 2. The best result is provided by our approach. In addition, as a no ROI dependent approach, our method detected all lymphomas comparing to the ground truth. Although it exists a certain quantity of false positive lymphomas (with average of $VOLUME_{sup} = 32\%$), our result is encouraging, shown in the Fig. 4. In Fig. 4 (a), the patient contains one lymphoma with high contrast of metabolism. Our method can well detect and segment it. Figure 4 (b) shows two lymphomas sites that have been detected and well segmented. The high metabolism area (heart) on the right corner had been removed by anatomical atlas, thus, no false positive detected regions. The situation is complex in Fig. 4 (c) because of a several sites similar to the lymphoma, our method obtained some false positive regions which can be removed by the user in the last step.

Table 2. Comparison results [2]

Approach name	Mean $DICE_{ref}$	Min $DICE_{ref}$	Max $DICE_{ref}$
40% SUVmax	72.9 ± 11.5	50.2	88.5
Black [8]	78.1 ± 9.4	58.4	89.6
Nestle [9]	78.9 ± 6.3	66.1	89.6
Vauclin [10]	72.2 ± 11.9	46.6	88.3
Fitting [2]	80.6 ± 4.7	68.9	88.4
CA [2]	80.0 ± 4.8	71.2	87.4
CRFs	**81.2 ± 11.8**	**61.2**	**95.9**

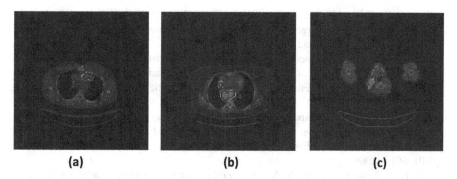

Fig. 4. Visualization of lymphoma segmentation on three different patients (a)(b)(c). Yellow contours are the manual references and blue contours are our results. (Color figure online)

4   Conclusion and Perspectives

Our approach applies an anatomical multi-atlas segmentation on the CT of the PET/CT to remove on the PET images the organs having physiological hyper metabolism and which are usually not concerned by the lymphoma (brain, heard, kidneys and bladder). Then a CRFs algorithm is developed for lymphoma detection and segmentation using medical knowledge and mathematical models for conditional probability. Finally, users can manually select lymphomas from the detected 3D regions. In future, more patients will be tested and a combination of PET and CT images will be considered to extend the unary energy.

References

1. Zaidi, H., El Naqa, I.: PET-guided delineation of radiation therapy treatment volumes: a survey of image segmentation techniques. Eur. J. Nucl. Med. Mol. Imaging **37**, 2165–2187 (2010)
2. Desbordes, P., Petitjean, C., Ruan, S.: 3D automated lymphoma segmentation in PET images based on cellular automata. IEEE, (2015). Electronic ISSN:2154-512X
3. Eloïse, G., Hugues, T., Nicolas, P., Michel, M., Laurent, N.: Automated 3D lymphoma lesion segmentation from PET/CT characteristics. In: Symposium on Biomedical Imaging: From Nano to Macro, pp. 174–178 (2017)
4. Shotton, J., Winn, J., Rother, C., Criminisi, A.: TextonBoost for image understanding: multi-class object recognition and segmentation by jointly modeling texture, layout, and context. Int. J. Comput. Vis. **81**, 2–23 (2007)
5. Krähenbühl, P., Koltun, V.: Efficient inference in fully connected CRFs with gaussian edge potentials. Adv. Neural. Inf. Process. Syst. **24**, 109–117 (2011)
6. Boykov, Y.Y., Jolly, M.-P.: Interactive graph cuts for optimal boundary and region segmentation of objects in N-D images. IEEE (2011). doi:10.1109/ICCV.2001.937505
7. Krähenbühl, P., Koltun, V.: Parameter learning and convergent inference for dense random fields. In: International Conference on Machine Learning (ICML) (2013)

8. Black, Q.C., Grills, I.S., Kestin, L.L., Wong, C.Y., Wong, J.W., Martinez, A.A., Yan, D.: Defining a radiotherapy target with positron emission tomography. Int. J. Radiat. Oncol. Biol. Phys. **60**(4), 1272–1282 (2004)
9. Nestle, U., Kremp, S., Schaefer-Schuler, A., Sebastian-Welsch, C., Hellwig, D., Rübe, C., Kirsch, C.M.: Comparison of different methods for delineation of 18F-FDG PET-positive tissue for target volume definition in radiotherapy of patients with non-Small cell lung cancer. J. Nucl. Med. **46**(8), 1342–1348 (2005)
10. Vauclin, S., Doyeux, K., Hapdey, S., Edet-Sanson, A., Vera, P., Gardin, I.: Development of a generic thresholding algorithm for the delineation of 18FDG-PET-positive tissue: application to the comparison of three thresholding models. Phys. Med. Biol. **54**(22), 6901–6916 (2009)
11. Rother, C., Kolmogorov, V., Blake, A.: GrabCut -interactive foreground extraction using iterated graph cuts. ACM Trans. Graph. (SIGGRAPH) (2004)
12. Yan, T., Liu, Q., Wei, Q., Chen, F., Deng, T.: Classification of lymphoma cell image based on improved SVM. In: Zhang, T.-C., Nakajima, M. (eds.) Advances in Applied Biotechnology. LNEE, vol. 332, pp. 199–208. Springer, Heidelberg (2015). doi:10.1007/978-3-662-45657-6_21
13. Sharif, M.S., Amira, A., Zaidi, H.: 3D oncological PET volume analysis using CNN and LVQNN. In: Circuits and Systems (ISCAS), Proceedings of 2010 IEEE International Symposium on Circuits and Systems: Nano-Bio Circuit Fabrics and Systems (ISCAS 2010), pp. 1783–1786, June 2010
14. Zhoubing, X.U., Ryan, R.P., Lee, C.P., Baucom, R.B., Poulose, B.K., Abramson, R.G., Landman, B.A.: Efficient multi-atlas abdominal segmentation on clinically acquired CT with SIMPLE context learning. Med. Image Anal. **24**(1), 18–27 (2015)
15. Tylski, P., Stute, S., Grotus, N., Doyeux, K., Hepdey, S., Gardin, I., Vanderlinden, B., Buvat, I.: Comparative assessment of methods for estimating tumor volume and standardized uptake value in (18) F-FDG PET. J. Nucl. Med. **51**, 268–276 (2010)
16. Szeliski, R., Zabih, R., Scharstein, D., Veksler, O., Kolmogorov, V., Agarwala, A., Tappen, M., Rother, C.A.: comparative study of energy minimization methods for Markov random fields with smoothness-based priors. IEEE Trans. Pattern Anal. Mach. Intell. **30**(6), 1068–1080 (2008)
17. Weiler-Sagie, M., Bushelev, O., Epelbaum, R., Dann, E.J., Haim, N., Avivi, I., Ben-Barak, A., Ben-Arie, Y., Bar-Shalom, R., Israel, O.: (18) F-FDG avidity in lymphoma readdressed: a study of 766 patients. J. Nucl. Med. **51**(1), 25–30 (2009)
18. Cottereau, A.-S., Lanic, H., Mareschal, S., Meignan, M., Vera, P., Tilly, H., Jardin, F., Becker, S.: Molecular profile and FDG-PET/CT total metabolic tumor volume improve risk classification at diagnosis for patients with diffuse large b-cell lymphoma. Clin. Cancer Res. **22**(15), 3801–3809 (2016)
19. Meignan, M., Sasanelli, M., Casasnovas, R.O., Luminari, S., Fioroni, F., Coriani, C., Masset, H., Itti, E., Gobbi, P.G., Merli, F., Versari, A.: Metabolic tumour volumes measured at staging in lymphoma: methodological evaluation on phantom experiments and patients. Eur. J. Nucl. Med. Mol. Imaging **41**(6), 1113–1122 (2014)
20. Meignan, M., Gallamini, A., Meignan, M., Gallamini, A., Haioun, C.: Report on the first international workshop on interim-PET scan in lymphoma. Leuk. Lymphoma **50**(8), 1257–1260 (2009)
21. Barrington, S.F., Kluge, R.: FDG PET for therapy monitoring in Hodgkin and non-Hodgkin lymphomas. Eur. J. Nucl. Med. Mol. Imaging (2017). doi:10.1007/s00259-017-3690-8

Individual Analysis of Molecular Brain Imaging Data Through Automatic Identification of Abnormality Patterns

Ninon Burgos[1,2(✉)], Jorge Samper-González[1,2], Anne Bertrand[1,2,3],
Marie-Odile Habert[4], Sébastien Ourselin[5,6], Stanley Durrleman[1,2],
M. Jorge Cardoso[5,6], and Olivier Colliot[1,2,3,7]

[1] Inria Paris, Aramis Project-Team, Paris, France
ninon.burgos@inria.fr
[2] Sorbonne Universités, UPMC Univ Paris 06, Inserm, CNRS,
Institut du Cerveau et la Moelle épinière (ICM) - Pitié-Salpêtrière Hospital,
Paris, France
[3] AP-HP, Department of Neuroradiology, Pitié-Salpêtrière Hospital, Paris, France
[4] AP-HP, Department of Nuclear Medicine, Sorbonne Universités,
Pitié-Salpêtrière Hospital, UPMC Univ Paris 06, Inserm U 1146,CNRS UMR 7371,
UMR 7371, Laboratoire d'Imagerie Biomédicale, Paris, France
[5] Translational Imaging Group, CMIC, University College London, London, UK
[6] Dementia Research Centre, University College London, London, UK
[7] AP-HP, Department of Neurology, Pitié-Salpêtrière Hospital, Paris, France

Abstract. We introduce a pipeline for the individual analysis of positron emission tomography (PET) data on large cohorts of patients. This pipeline consists for each individual of generating a subject-specific model of healthy PET appearance and comparing the individual's PET image to the model via a novel regularised Z-score. The resulting voxel-wise Z-score map can be interpreted as a subject-specific abnormality map that summarises the pathology's topographical distribution in the brain. We then propose a strategy to validate the abnormality maps on several PET tracers and automatically detect the underlying pathology by using the abnormality maps as features to feed a linear support vector machine (SVM)-based classifier.

We applied the pipeline to a large dataset comprising 298 subjects selected from the ADNI2 database (103 cognitively normal, 105 late MCI and 90 Alzheimer's disease subjects). The high classification accuracy obtained when using the abnormality maps as features demonstrates that the proposed pipeline is able to extract for each individual the signal characteristic of dementia from both FDG and Florbetapir PET data.

1 Introduction

Long before the clinical symptoms of the disease appear, neuroimaging, mainly magnetic resonance (MR) and positron emission tomography (PET), plays an important role in the diagnosis of dementia [1]. Information derived from PET

© Springer International Publishing AG 2017
M.J. Cardoso et al. (Eds.): CMMI/RAMBO/SWITCH 2017, LNCS 10555, pp. 13–22, 2017.
DOI: 10.1007/978-3-319-67564-0_2

images is of crucial value: ^{18}F-fluorodeoxyglucose (FDG) PET reflects the glucose consumption, which correlates with the activity of the synapses, while other PET tracers such as Florbetapir are used to image the deposition of beta-amyloid (Aβ) plaques in the brain. However, the analysis of multiple imaging modalities for diagnostic purposes is to date challenging, and hardly translated to clinical practice. The main drawback is represented by the large amount of information that needs to be consistently processed and analysed to derive clinically useful information.

A popular way to extract meaningful information from neurological images is to use computational methods based on machine learning to directly estimate the category of pathology in a patient. Most machine learning methods developed for classification in dementia studies extract the features used to draw the border that differentiates normality from abnormality directly from the images, e.g. thickness of the cortex extracted from structural MR images [2], or glucose consumption extracted from PET images [3]. However, these features are affected by the anatomical variability present in the population, which acts as a confounding factor making the task of finding the frontier (i.e. the decision function) between normality and abnormality very challenging. Instead of trying to find this frontier at the population level, transporting the problem to the individual level might reduce its complexity.

In previous work, we developed a framework for the analysis of FDG PET data that consists of creating a patient-specific model of healthy PET appearance and comparing the patient's PET image to the model via a Z-score, thus providing voxel-wise statistics on the variation of glucose metabolism in a control population [4]. We showed that this approach was able to distinguish subgroups in a small dataset comprising 22 subjects with distinct neurodegenerative syndromes [4].

In this paper, we introduce a pipeline for the individual analysis of PET data on large cohorts of patients. This pipeline consists of generating a subject-specific model of healthy PET appearance for each subject following the method described in [4] and comparing the subject's PET image to the model via a novel regularised Z-score, which results in the generation of subject-specific abnormality maps summarising the pathology's topographical distribution in the brain. We then propose a strategy to validate the abnormality maps on several PET tracers and automatically detect dementia by using the abnormality maps as features to feed a linear support vector machine (SVM)-based classifier. This strategy enables us to assess on a large dataset composed of 298 subjects selected from the ADNI2 database if the proposed subject-specific abnormality maps are able to extract for each individual the signal characteristic of abnormality from both FDG and Florbetapir PET data, with the aim to reduce the confounding impact of anatomical variability when trying to distinguish disease versus normal ageing.

2   Methods

2.1   Data

Imaging data were obtained from the ADNI2 database[1]. We selected 298 participants who had T1-weighted MRI, ^{18}F-FDG PET, and Florbetapir (^{18}F-AV45) PET images at baseline and were diagnosed as cognitively normal (CN) (n = 103, 68 Aβ^-), late mild cognitive impairment (LMCI) (n = 105, 71 Aβ^+) or Alzheimer's disease (AD) (n = 90, 80 Aβ^+). In [5], Landau et al. categorised subjects as amyloid positive (Aβ^+) or negative (Aβ^-) on Florbetapir based on a cortical mean cutoff of 1.11. Here, we define as amyloid positive the subjects with a cortical mean standardised uptake value ratio (SUVR) higher than $1.11 + 5\%$ and as amyloid negative the subjects with a cortical mean SUVR lower than $1.11 - 5\%$. The control dataset used in this paper is composed of the CN participants amyloid negative (n = 68).

2.2   Data Preprocessing

PET images were downloaded from the ADNI website after pre-processing (frame averaging, spatial alignment, interpolation to a standard voxel size, and smoothing to a common resolution of 8 mm full width at half maximum). For each subject, the T1 image was mapped to the PET images using a rigid transformation. The T1 images from all the subjects were then mapped to a common coordinate frame via an affine groupwise registration [6]. Finally, the transformations were applied to the T1, FDG PET and AV45 PET images by updating their image coordinate system (without resampling), forming a database of T1 and PET images globally aligned in a common space.

2.3   Subject-Specific Analysis of PET Data

The proposed subject-specific PET analysis framework consisted of selecting in the control dataset the subjects that were morphologically the most similar to the subject being analysed, creating subject-specific models of healthy PET uptake from the selected controls and the target subject's T1 image, and using the resulting model to create subject-specific abnormality maps.

Selection Based on Global and Local Image Similarity Measures. Subjects were first selected from the control dataset according to their global morphological similarity to the target subject, as assessed by a global similarity measure, the normalised cross-correlation (NCC). Because all the subjects were pre-aligned with each other, the T1 image of each subjects was simply resampled to the common space and the NCC was computed between each resampled control subject and the resampled target subject. The 50 control subjects with

---

[1] Imaging data were provided by the Alzheimer's disease neuroimaging initiative (http://adni.loni.ucla.edu/).

the highest NCC were selected (top 75%). This step is meant to discard the controls too dissimilar to the target and thus limit the computational time while maintaining a high synthesis accuracy.

The T1 images of the 50 pre-selected controls were then non-rigidly registered to the target subject's T1 image in its native space [7], and the PET images of the control dataset, pre-aligned to the T1 images, were mapped using the same transformation to the target subject. Once non-rigidly aligned to the target subject, the controls morphologically the most similar to the target subject at the voxel level were identified using a local image similarity measure, the structural image similarity (SSIM) [8].

Subject-Specific Models of Healthy PET Appearance. To generate the subject-specific model, which is composed of two elements: a spatially-varying weighted average and a spatially-varying weighted standard deviation, the controls locally selected were fused based on their morphological similarity to the target subject. The weights, corresponding to the contribution of each control subject to the model, were obtained by ranking at each voxel x the SSIM across the N globally pre-selected control subjects and applying an exponential decay function: $w_n(x) = e^{-\beta r_n(x)}$, where $r_n(x)$ denotes the rank of the nth control subject, and $\beta = 0.5$ [4]. For each of the N pre-selected subjects in the control dataset, let the nth mapped PET image be denoted by J_n. The two subject-specific model elements (I_μ, I_σ) are computed as follows:

$$I_\mu(x) = \frac{\sum_{n=1}^{N} w_n(x) \cdot J_n(x)}{\sum_{n=1}^{N} w_n(x)} \quad ,$$

$$I_\sigma(x) = \sqrt{\frac{N_w}{N_w - 1} \frac{\sum_{n=1}^{N} w_n(x) \cdot (J_n(x) - I_\mu(x))^2}{\sum_{n=1}^{N} w_n(x)}}$$

$$(1)$$

where N_w is the number of non-zero weights.

Subject-Specific Abnormality Maps. To compare the target subject's PET image to the subject-specific model, in [4] a Z-score was computed for each voxel of the image. However, we observed that this leads to the generation of high frequency signals in certain areas due to the standard deviation approaching zero. To avoid this problem, we define a regularised Z-score

$$\tilde{Z}(x) = \frac{I(x) - I_\mu(x)}{I_\sigma(x) + \alpha * I_{\bar{\sigma}}} \tag{2}$$

where $I_{\bar{\sigma}}$ is the standard deviation averaged over all the voxels. We set α equal to 2 as a compromise between the resulting Z-score maps being too smooth and the presence of high frequency signals. The voxel-wise regularised Z-score map can be interpreted as an *abnormality map*, as it statistically evaluates the localised deviation of the subject-specific uptake with respect to the healthy uptake distribution.

2.4   Validation Scheme

To assess the ability of the abnormality maps to extract relevant information from PET data on a large dataset and to offer a new strategy for computer-assisted diagnosis, we propose to use the abnormality maps as features to feed a linear SVM classifier.

Non-linear Alignment to Group Space. A way to compare the abnormality maps, each generated in the subject's native space, across all the subjects, is to align them with each other. As the T1 images from all the subjects were already mapped to a common coordinate frame via an affine groupwise registration, the T1 images were subsequently non-rigidly registered to the group-space. The same transformations were then applied to the abnormality maps.

Linear SVM Classifier. We chose a linear SVM to classify the abnormality maps. A linear kernel was calculated using the inner product for each pair of abnormality maps available in the dataset (using all the brain voxels). This kernel was then used as input for the generic SVM[2]. Two nested 10-fold cross-validation procedures were used to train the classifier and to optimise the hyperparameters. The process was repeated ten times and the classification results averaged over the ten repeats. This process guarantees an unbiased evaluation of the classification accuracy.

Classification Tasks. The experiments consisted of two simple tasks:

1. differentiating cognitively normal subjects from subjects with a disease, i.e. CN vs AD and CN vs LMCI;
2. differentiating between amyloid negative and amyloid positive subjects (β^- vs β^+).

For the first experiment, 219 subjects (68 CN $A\beta^-$, 71 LMCI $A\beta^+$ and 80 AD $A\beta^+$) were considered, while for the second experiment 298 subjects (112 $A\beta^-$ and 186 $A\beta^+$) were analysed.

Comparison to State-of-the-Art. To set the results in perspective, the subjects' PET images themselves and state-of-the-art Z-maps were also used as features and fed to the classifier. The state-of-the-art Z-maps were obtained by comparing the subject's PET image in the group space to the mean and standard deviation computed from all the 68 subjects in the control dataset, also in the group space.

---

[2] http://scikit-learn.org.

3   Results

Abnormality maps were generated for each of the 298 ADNI2 participants selected, for both the FDG and AV45 PET images. Note that for the CN β^- subjects (forming the control dataset), a leave-one-out strategy was used, i.e. the images of the CN subject being processed were excluded from the control database. Examples of abnormality maps are displayed in Fig. 1 for a CN, a late MCI and an AD subject. We observe that, as expected, no specific signal is being detected for the CN subject, for both the FDG and AV45 tracers. For the LMCI subject, abnormal glucose uptake is detected mainly in the precuneus and in the cingulate gyrus, and abnormal amyloid deposition is detected in the frontal, parietal, temporal and cingulate cortices, which is consistent with previous

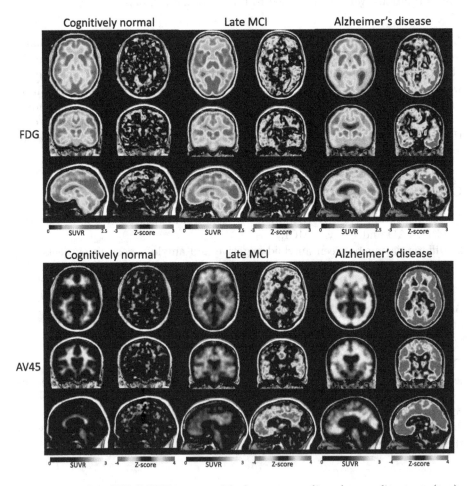

Fig. 1. Examples of FDG PET images with the corresponding abnormality maps (top) and of AV45 PET images with the corresponding abnormality maps (bottom) for a CN, an LMCI and an AD subject.

Table 1. Balanced accuracy obtained when using PET images, state-of-the-art Z-maps, and the proposed subject-specific abnormality maps as features of the linear SVM classification algorithm. The average ± SD balanced accuracy, obtained over ten repeats, is expressed in percentages.

	FDG			AV45		
	PET	Zmap	Abn. map	PET	Zmap	Abn. map
CN vs AD	88.9 ± 1.1	89.6 ± 1.2	91.6 ± 1.2	100 ± 0	100 ± 0	100 ± 0
CN vs LMCI	78.3 ± 1.7	78.7 ± 1.9	80.5 ± 1.6	100 ± 0	100 ± 0	99.5 ± 0.5
$A\beta^+$ vs $A\beta^-$	71.5 ± 1.0	71.4 ± 1.1	73.9 ± 1.7	99.8 ± 0.4	99.4 ± 0.5	99.7 ± 0.5

observations [9]. Finally, for the AD subject, abnormal glucose uptake is detected in areas such as the hypocampus, the precuneus, the cingulate gyrus or the occipital cortex, and abnormal amyloid deposition is detected in all the cortex, which is typical of AD [1].

The abnormality maps were then fed to the linear SVM classifier. The balanced accuracy obtained with the proposed method applied to the FDG data when differentiating CN from AD and LMCI (92% and 81%, respectively) is higher than the balanced accuracy obtained using PET SUVR values (89% and 78%) and the state-of-the-art Z-maps (90% and 79%) as features. Similar results were obtained when differentiating amyloid negative and positive subjects. When analysing AV45 data, using the PET images themselves, the state-of-the-art Z-maps or the proposed abnormality maps leads to similar, highly accurate, classification results. These highly accurate results were expected, but are here confirmed, as differentiating CN ($A\beta^-$) from AD and LMCI (both $A\beta^+$) subjects, or amyloid negative from amyloid positive subjects, based on features extracted from AV45 data is a quite trivial task. More detailed results are shown in Table 1. The high classification accuracy obtained with the abnormality maps confirms their ability to detect meaningful signal from both FDG and AV45 PET images.

To further analyse the classification results, we studied the feature maps generated by the linear SVM classifier that show which voxels are relevant for each classification task. The maps obtained for the classification of CN vs AD subjects and CN vs LMCI subjects are shown in Fig. 2. We observe that the areas that were detected as abnormal with the proposed method (i.e. hypocampus, precuneus, cingulate gyrus) are also the ones mostly used to separate AD from CN subjects, no matter the features used. We also observe that these areas are more strongly targeted when the abnormality maps are used as features compared to the PET images themselves or the state-of-the-art Zmaps. This confirms the ability of the abnormality maps to detect areas that are characteristic of AD. A similar trend was observed for the classification of CN vs LMCI subjects and for the classification of $A\beta^+$ vs $A\beta^-$ subjects (not shown).

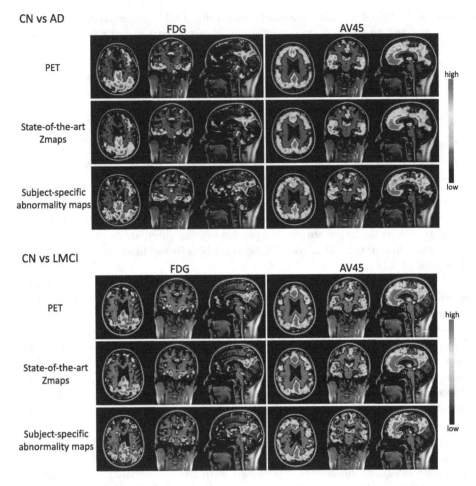

Fig. 2. Voxels the most relevant for the classification of CN vs AD (top) and CN vs LMCI (bottom) subjects when using the PET images themselves, the state-of-the-art Zmaps and the proposed subject-specific abnormality maps as features, for both the FDG and AV45 tracers. The red areas indicate the regions that are mostly used to separate AD or LMCI from CN subjects. (Color figure online)

4   Discussion and Conclusion

This paper presents a pipeline for the individual analysis of molecular brain images on large-scale datasets. This pipeline is able to automatically locate and characterise the areas characteristic of dementia by generating abnormality maps summarising the pathology's topographical distribution in the brain. This ability was demonstrated by using the abnormality maps as inputs of a classifier and comparing the classification results to the ones obtained when using the PET images themselves or state-of-the art Z-maps as features. Although the three methods produced a high classification accuracy when differentiating CN from late MCI and AD, and when differentiating amyloid negative subjects from amyloid positive subjects, more accurate results were obtained with the proposed method. These results can be explained by the fact that both the PET images and the state-of-the-art Z-maps are affected by the anatomical variability present in the population, which acts as a confounding factor when trying to differentiate between normality and abnormality. As the subject-specific mean and standard deviation used to compute the abnormality maps are obtained by selecting the subjects in the control dataset that are morphologically the most similar to target subject, the abnormality maps are less impacted by morphological variability.

The abnormality maps have two complementary uses. They can (i) help clinicians in their diagnosis by highlighting, in a data-driven fashion, the pathological areas obtained from the individual PET data, and (ii) provide quantitative, voxel-based, abnormality scores that can be used as input for computer-assisted diagnosis tools for the automatic detection of dementia.

Acknowledgements. The research leading to these results has received funding from the People Programme (Marie Curie Actions) of the European Union's Seventh Framework Programme (FP7/2007-2013) under REA grant agreement no. PCOFUND-GA-2013-609102, through the PRESTIGE programme coordinated by Campus France, and from the programme "Investissements d'avenir" ANR-10-IAIHU-06.

References

1. Jagust, W.: Positron emission tomography and magnetic resonance imaging in the diagnosis and prediction of dementia. Alzheimer's Dement. **2**(1), 36–42 (2006)
2. Klöppel, S., Stonnington, C.M., Chu, C., Draganski, B., Scahill, R.I., Rohrer, J.D., Fox, N.C., Jack, C.R., Ashburner, J., Frackowiak, R.S.: Automatic classification of MR scans in Alzheimer's disease. Brain **131**(3), 681–689 (2008)
3. Illán, I., Górriz, J., Ramírez, J., Salas-Gonzalez, D., López, M., Segovia, F., Chaves, R., Gómez-Rio, M., Puntonet, C.G.: The Alzheimer's disease neuroimaging initiative: ^{18}F-FDG PET imaging analysis for computer aided Alzheimer's diagnosis. Inf. Sci. **181**(4), 903–916 (2011)
4. Burgos, N., Jorge Cardoso, M., Mendelson, A.F., Schott, J.M., Atkinson, D., Arridge, S.R., Hutton, B.F., Ourselin, S.: Subject-specific models for the analysis of pathological FDG PET data. In: Navab, N., Hornegger, J., Wells, W.M., Frangi, A.F. (eds.) MICCAI 2015. LNCS, vol. 9350, pp. 651–658. Springer, Cham (2015). doi:10.1007/978-3-319-24571-3_78
5. Landau, S.M., Mintun, M.A., Joshi, A.D., Koeppe, R.A., Petersen, R.C., Aisen, P.S., Weiner, M.W., Jagust, W.J.: Amyloid deposition, hypometabolism, and longitudinal cognitive decline. Ann. Neurol. **72**(4), 578–586 (2012)
6. Modat, M., Cash, D.M., Daga, P., Winston, G.P., Duncan, J.S., Ourselin, S.: A symmetric block-matching framework for global registration. In: Proceedings of SPIE, Medical Imaging, vol. 9034 (2014)
7. Modat, M., Ridgway, G.R., Taylor, Z.A., Lehmann, M., Barnes, J., Hawkes, D.J., Fox, N.C., Ourselin, S.: Fast free-form deformation using graphics processing units. Comput. Methods Programs Biomed. **98**(3), 278–84 (2010)

8. Wang, Z., Bovik, A.C., Sheikh, H.R., Simoncelli, E.P.: Image quality assessment: from error visibility to structural similarity. IEEE Trans. Image Process. **13**(4), 600–612 (2004)
9. Forsberg, A., Engler, H., Almkvist, O., Blomquist, G., Hagman, G., Wall, A., Ringheim, A., Långström, B., Nordberg, A.: PET imaging of amyloid deposition in patients with mild cognitive impairment. Neurobiol. Aging **29**(10), 1456–1465 (2008)

W-Net for Whole-Body Bone Lesion Detection on ^{68}Ga-Pentixafor PET/CT Imaging of Multiple Myeloma Patients

Lina Xu[1,3]($\boxtimes$), Giles Tetteh[1,2], Mona Mustafa[3], Jana Lipkova[1,2], Yu Zhao[1,2], Marie Bieth[1,2], Patrick Christ[1,2], Marie Piraud[1,2], Bjoern Menze[1,2], and Kuangyu Shi[3]

[1] Department of Computer Science, TU München, Munich, Germany
lina.xu@tum.de
[2] Institute of Medical Engineering, TU München, Munich, Germany
[3] Department of Nuclear Medicine, Klinikum Rechts der Isar, TU München, Munich, Germany

Abstract. The assessment of bone lesion is crucial for the diagnostic and therapeutic planning of multiple myeloma (MM). ^{68}Ga-Pentixafor PET/CT can capture the abnormal molecular expression of CXCR-4 in addition to anatomical changes. However, the whole-body detection of dozens of lesions on hybrid imaging is tedious and error-prone. In this paper, we adopt a cascaded convolutional neural networks (CNN) to form a W-shaped architecture (W-Net). This deep learning method leverages multimodal information for lesion detection. The first part of W-Net extracts skeleton from CT scan and the second part detect and segment lesions. The network was tested on 12 ^{68}Ga-Pentixafor PET/CT scans of MM patients using 3-folder cross validation. The preliminary results showed that W-Net can automatically learn features from multimodal imaging for MM bone lesion detection. The proof-of-concept study encouraged further development of deep learning approach for MM lesion detection with increased number of subjects.

1 Introduction

Multiple myeloma (MM) is a type of hematological malignancy with the proliferation of neoplasma cells in the bone marrow [1]. It accounts for 13% of all hematologic malignancies and 1% of all malignancies [2]. Common symptoms of MM are summarized as CRAB: hypercalcemia (C), renal failure (R), anemia (A), and bone lesions (B). Modern treatment has achieved a 5-year survival rate of 45% [3]. Nevertheless, MM remains an incurable disease at the moment and it usually relapses after a period of remission over therapy. The identification of bone lesions plays an important role in the diagnostic and therapeutic assessment of MM.

L. Xu and G. Tetteh—Contributed equally to this work.

© Springer International Publishing AG 2017
M.J. Cardoso et al. (Eds.): CMMI/RAMBO/SWITCH 2017, LNCS 10555, pp. 23–30, 2017.
DOI: 10.1007/978-3-319-67564-0_3

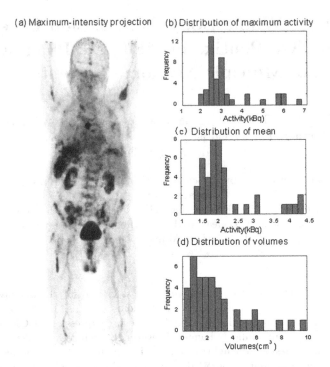

(a) Maximum-intensity projection   (b) Distribution of maximum activity

(c) Distribution of mean

(d) Distribution of volumes

Fig. 1. Properties of MM lesions of an exemplary patient with ^{68}Ga-Pentixafor PET imaging: (a) maximum-intensity projection of ^{68}Ga-Pentixafor PET; (b) histogram distribution of maximum activity of the lesions; (c) histogram distribution of mean activity of the lesions; (d) histogram distribution of volumes of the lesions.

Traditional radiographic skeletal survey (whole body X-ray), which is widely used, is limited in sensitivity and detection accuracy. It can only sense lesions when the trabecular bone has already lost more than 30% [4]. 3D computed tomography (CT) allows the detection of smaller bone lesions that are not detectable by conventional radiography [5]. Magnetic resonance imaging (MRI) is also more sensitive than skeletal survey in the detection of MM lesions and it can detect diffuse bone marrow infiltration [6]. Comparable high sensitivity in the detection of small bone lesions can be achieved using PET/CT by combining metabolic (^{18}F-FDG PET) and anatomical (CT) information [7,8]. The lesions can be visualized more clearly with the guidance of hotspots in fused images. Recently the overexpression of chemokine (C-X-C motif) receptor 4 (CXCR4) has been verified in a variety of cancers, leading to the development of targeted PET tracer such as ^{68}Ga-Pentixafor [9]. This emerging tracer has already demonstrated higher sensitivity in the visualization of MM lesions [10]. Even though, systematically detecting bone lesions remains problematic due to the heterogeneous size and uptake. Manual evaluation can result in variability between different observers [11] and may be prone to errors. As is shown in Fig. 1, the ^{68}Ga-Pentixafor PET imaging has a large variation in uptake and size even among the lesions in the same patient. Such heterogeneity in the complex context with various unspecific uptake makes the whole-body detection of all the lesions extremely difficult. So far, no effective methods has been presented for automated detection of these MM bone lesions.

Computer-aided detection (CAD) has been developed to assist radiologists to resolve the critical information from complex data, which improves the accuracy and robustness of diagnosis [12–14]. Machine learning is the engine for typical CAD approaches [15]. Several methods have been developed to detect lesions in oncological applications [16], in which lesion and non-lesion parts are differentiated and segmented. Random walk and graph cut method were integrated for segmenting tumors in PET/CT scans [17]. A probabilistic, spatially dependent density model has been developed to automatically identify bone marrow infiltration for femur lesions in low-dose CT [18]. The convolutional neural network (CNN), such as U-Net, offers a 2D framework to segment biomedical images [19]. It is extended to a 3D version as V-Net [20] and achieves good results by introducing an optimized objective function to train the data end-to-end. A cascaded fully CNNs has been developed to first segment the liver and then the liver lesion [21].

In this paper, we aim to automatically detect MM lesions by taking advantage of both molecular and anatomical features from ^{68}Ga-Pentixafor PET/CT whole-body scans. Two enhanced V-nets are cascaded to build a W-shaped framework to learn the volumetric feature representation of the skeleton and its lesions from coarse to fine. The network does not require the extraction of features for learning. The proposed method is trained and tested on 12 patients diagnosed with MM and the preliminary results demonstrate its potential to improve the MM bone lesion detection.

2   Method and Experiment

2.1   Data Preparation and Preprocessing

A total of 12 patients (3 female and 9 male) with histologically proven multiple myeloma disease were referred for ^{68}Ga-Pentixafor PET/CT imaging (Siemens Biograph mCT 64; Siemens Medical Solutions, Germany). Approximately 90 to 205 MBq 68Ga-Pentixafor was injected intravenously 1 h before the scan. A low-dose CT (20 mAs, 120 keV) covering the body from the base of skull to the proximal thighs was scanned for attenuation correction. PET emission data were acquired using a 3D mode with a 200×200 matrix for around 3 min emission time per bed position. PET data were corrected for decay and scattering and iteratively reconstructed with attenuation correction. This study was approved by the corresponding ethics committees. Patients were given written informed consent prior to the investigations. The co-registration of PET and CT were visually inspected using PMOD. With the fusion of PET and CT, all the lesions were manually annotated by an experienced senior radiologist. Then each lesion was segmented by local thresholding at half maximum using PMOD.

2.2 W-Net Deep Learning Architecture

A deep learning-based architecture is adopted for automated whole-body multiple myeloma bone lesion detection, which is implemented by segmenting the lesions inside the bone. We explore a popular CNN-based deep learning architecture, V-Net, for 3D volumetric image segmentation [20] on hybrid PET/CT scans. Two V-Nets are cacascaded to form a W-Net architecture to improve the segmentation to bone-specific lesions. As illustrated in Fig. 2, there is a compression downward path, followed by an approximately symmetry decompression path inside each V-Net. The former cuts the volumetric size and broadens the receptive field along the layers, while the latter functions the opposite to expand the spatial support of the lower resolution feature maps. For both contracting and expansive path, we use the same $3 \times 3 \times 3$ kernel for convolution and a stride of two for max pooling or up sampling. For the first one, only volumetric CT data is fed into the network in order to learn anatomical knowledge about the bone. The outcome builds a binary mask for the skeleton, which adaptively offers geometrical boundary for lesion localization. The second V-Net then adds both PET/CT and the output from the first network as the total input, of which PET/CT provides additional feature information to jointly predict the lesion.

The W-Net architecture and experiments are conducted on Theano and all the PET/CT volumes are trained on NVIDIA TITAN X with a GPU memory of 12 GB. We employed 3-fold cross validation to test the prediction accuracy. Dice score was calculated to estimate the segmentation accuracy. In addition, the lesion-wise detection accuracies (sensitivity, specification, precision) was summarized on the segmented results based on the criteria of bounding box overlap. The bounding boxes of size $9 \times 9 \times 9$ were generated across the lesions with an overlap of 4 voxels being added in all three directions. A lesion was considered as detected when the amount of lesion labels fell into the bounding box is above 10%.

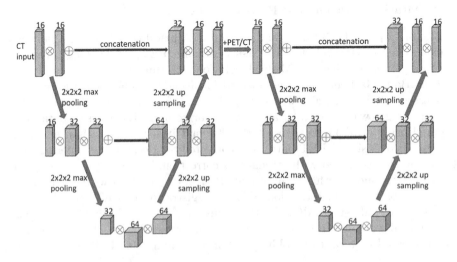

Fig. 2. Overview of a simplified W-Net architecture.

3   Results and Discussion

The performance of W-Net is trained and tested on ^{68}Ga-Pentixafor PET/CT scan of twelve MM patients. Exemplary detection results of 3 slices at different body regions are visualized in axial plane in Fig. 3, where the bone lesion segmentation is denoted in red. Yellow arrow represents false positive detection and false negatives are marked in green. Typically, false negative occurs when the lesion is too small while the contrast is not enough to identify its presence. The false positive is highly intensity driven, which considers the non-specific high tracer uptake as lesion by mistake. For W-Net, the obtained binary skeleton mask is forwarded to the second V-Net together with PET/CT volumes. Therefore, W-Net geometrically offers extra anatomical restrictions and reduces the probability of assigning wrong lesion labels.

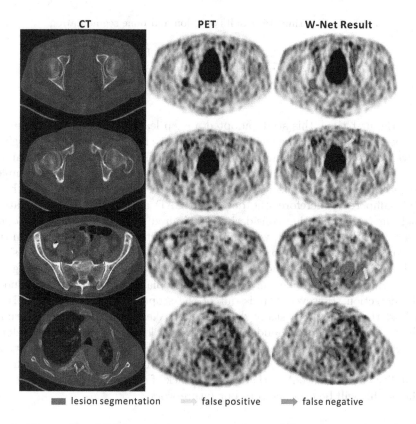

Fig. 3. Expemplary MM bone lesion segmentation and detection results. The first column gives the original CT scan in axial direction, the second column gives the corresponding PET scan and the third column shows MM bone lesion prediction using W-Net. (Color figure online)

Table 1 shows the performance of MM bone lesion detection. The W-Net, which combines PET/CT with additional binary skeletal mask, reaches a Dice score of 72.98%. It also obtains similar score for sensitivity (73.50%) and precision (72.46%). Besides distinguishing the information on CT and PET, and the extracted CT skeleton can be utilized for the regularization. The maximization of information utilization improves the segmentation and lesion detection. However, the overall performance of the W-Net may be restricted by the first V-Net. If the skeleton mask is not correctly labeled, its segmentation error will be propagated to the second V-Net and once again cause negative effect on lesion detection subsequently. Further improvement of the individual V-Net may improve the overall performance. In addition, W-Net obtains very high specificity (true negative rate) as 99.59%, which demonstrates the deep learning methods can properly exclude non-lesion parts.

Table 1. Experimental results of lesion and bone segmentation

Performance (%)	Sensitivity	Specificity	Precision	Dice
MM bone lesion	73.50%	99.59%	72.46%	72.98%

For the first time, this study adopted a deep learning method to automatically detect and segment the whole-body MM bone lesions on CXCR-4 imaging. However, it also has certain limitations as our work is restricted by small number of patient data. Even though we try to augment the number of training samples by generating bounding boxes, the performance of the deep learning methods is still hampered. Therefore, the developed CAD approach is yet not mature enough for real application considering the limited segmentation and detection accuracy. On the other hand, we only focus on multiple myeloma resided in the bone, for severe cases with bone marrow infiltration, where the myeloma lesions already outgrow from the bone structure and penetrate into the surrounding tissue (known as extramedullary myeloma), the neoplasma should be also included in the detection. However, this is out of the scope of our current goal. Nevertheless, this explorative study demonstrated the potential of deep learning methods in combining multimodal information for lesion detection. The preliminary results support the further development of deep learning methods for whole body lesion prediction. The performance is expected to be improved with the availability of more data. And there is also a lack of contrastive study with other methods, this will be conducted as our future work.

4   Conclusion

This paper employed a W-Net architecture to volumetrically learn and predict MM bone lesions on whole-body ^{68}Ga-Pentixafor PET/CT imaging. It explored a deep learning scheme for lesion segmentation and detection. The deep method does not require manual extraction of learning features. The preliminary results based on limited number of data support the W-Net with additional skeletal regularization for MM bone lesion detection. Increasing the data may further enhance the detection performance. The implementation of this study makes a step further towards developing an automated tool for multiple myeloma bone lesion detection.

References

1. Callander, N.S., Roodman, G.D.: Myeloma bone disease, pp. 276–285. Semin Hematol Elsevier (2001)
2. Collins, C.D.: Problems monitoring response in multiple myeloma. Cancer Imaging **5**, S119–S126 (2005)
3. Ltje, S., de Rooy, J.W., Croockewit, S., et al.: Role of radiography, MRI and FDG-PET/CT in diagnosing, staging and therapeutical evaluation of patients with multiple myeloma. Ann. Hematol. **88**, 1161–1168 (2009)
4. Dimopoulos, M., Terpos, E., Comenzo, R., et al.: International myeloma working group consensus statement and guidelines regarding the current role of imaging techniques in the diagnosis and monitoring of multiple Myeloma. Leukemia **23**, 1545–1556 (2009)
5. Horger, M., Claussen, C.D., Bross-Bach, U., et al.: Whole-body low-dose multidetector row-CT in the diagnosis of multiple myeloma: an alternative to conventional radiography. Eur. J. Radiol. **54**, 289–297 (2005)
6. Dutoit, J.C., Verstraete, K.L.: MRI in multiple myeloma: a pictorial review of diagnostic and post-treatment findings. Insights Image **7**, 553–569 (2016)
7. Healy, C.F., Murray, J.G., Eustace, S.J., et al.: Multiple myeloma: a review of imaging features and radiological techniques. Bone Marrow Res. (2011)
8. van Lammeren-Venema, D., Regelink, J.C., Riphagen, I.I., et al.: 18F-fluorodeoxyglucose positron emission tomography in assessment of myeloma-related bone disease: a systematic review. Cancer **118**(8), 1971–1981 (2012)
9. Vag, T., Gerngross, C., Herhaus, P., et al.: First experience with chemokine receptor CXCR4-targeted PET imaging of patients with solid cancers. J. Nucl. Med. **57**, 741–746 (2016)
10. Philipp-Abbrederis, K., Herrmann, K., Knop, S., et al.: In vivo molecular imaging of chemokine receptor CXCR4 expression in patients with advanced multiple myeloma. EMBO Mol. Med. (2015)
11. Belton, A., Saini, S., Liebermann, K., et al.: Tumour size measurement in an oncology clinical trial: comparison between off-site and on-site measurements. Clin. Radiol. **58**, 311–314 (2003)
12. Eadie, L.H., Taylor, P., Gibson, A.P.: A systematic review of computer-assisted diagnosis in diagnostic cancer imaging. Eur. J. Radiol. **81**, e70–e76 (2012)
13. Petrick, N., Sahiner, B., Armato, S.G., et al.: Evaluation of computer-aided detection and diagnosis systems. Med. Phys. **40**(8) (2013)
14. Taylor, A.T., Garcia, E.V.: Computer-assisted diagnosis in renal nuclear medicine: rationale, methodology, and interpretative criteria for diuretic renography. Semin. Nucl. Med. **44**, 146–158 (2014)
15. Wang, S., Summers, R.M.: Machine learning and radiology. Med. Image Anal. **16**, 933–951 (2012)

16. Kourou, K., Exarchos, T.P., Exarchos, K.P., et al.: Machine learning applications in cancer prognosis and prediction. Comput. Struct. Biotechnol. J. **13**, 8–17 (2015)

17. Ju, W., Xiang, D., Zhang, B., et al.: Random walk and graph cut for co-segmentation of lung tumor on PET-CT images. IEEE Trans. Med. Imaging **24**(12), 5854–5867 (2015)

18. Martínez-Martínez, F., Kybic, J., Lambert, L., et al.: Fully automated classification of bone marrow infiltration in low-dose CT of patients with multiple myeloma based on probabilistic density model and supervised learning. Comput. Biol. Med. **71**, 57–66 (2016)

19. Ronneberger, O., Fischer, P., Brox, T.: U-net: convolutional networks for biomedical image segmentation. In: Navab, N., Hornegger, J., Wells, W.M., Frangi, A.F. (eds.) MICCAI 2015. LNCS, vol. 9351, pp. 234–241. Springer, Cham (2015). doi:10. 1007/978-3-319-24574-4_28

20. Milletari, F., Navab, N., Ahmadi, S.A.: V-net: fully convolutional neural networks for volumetric medical image segmentation. In: 3DV, pp. 565–571 (2016)

21. Christ, P.F., et al.: Automatic liver and lesion segmentation in CT using cascaded fully convolutional neural networks and 3D conditional random fields. In: Ourselin, S., Joskowicz, L., Sabuncu, M.R., Unal, G., Wells, W. (eds.) MICCAI 2016. LNCS, vol. 9901, pp. 415–423. Springer, Cham (2016). doi:10.1007/978-3-319-46723-8_48

3D Alpha Matting Based Co-segmentation of Tumors on PET-CT Images

Zisha Zhong[1(✉)], Yusung Kim[2], John Buatti[2], and Xiaodong Wu[1,2]

[1] Department of Electrical and Computer Engineering, University of Iowa,
4016 Seamans Center, Iowa City, IA 52242, USA
zisha-zhong@uiowa.edu
[2] Department of Radiation Oncology, University of Iowa, 200 Hawkins Drive,
Iowa City, IA 52242, USA

Abstract. Positron emission tomography – computed tomography (PET-CT) has been widely used in modern cancer imaging. Accurate tumor delineation from PET and CT plays an important role in radiation therapy. The PET-CT co-segmentation technique, which makes use of advantages of both modalities, has achieved impressive performance for tumor delineation. In this work, we propose a novel 3D image matting based semi-automated co-segmentation method for tumor delineation on dual PET-CT scans. The "matte" values generated by 3D image matting are employed to compute the region costs for the graph based co-segmentation. Compared to previous PET-CT co-segmentation methods, our method is completely data-driven in the design of cost functions, thus using much less hyper-parameters in our segmentation model. Comparative experiments on 54 PET-CT scans of lung cancer patients demonstrated the effectiveness of our method.

Keywords: Image segmentation · Interactive segmentation · Lung tumor segmentation · Image matting · Co-segmentation

1 Introduction

Positron emission tomography – computed tomography (PET-CT) has revolutionized modern cancer imaging. Improved determination of the extent of cancer spread (staging) in patients by PET has illustrated the compelling need of acquiring this information for determining the therapeutic method to achieve improved prognoses. The integrated PET-CT, by adding precise anatomic localization to functional imaging, currently provides the most sensitive and accurate information available on tumor extent and distribution for a variety of common cancers. It increasingly plays a critically important role in tumor staging, clinical management/decision making, treatment planning, and therapy response assessment [1–3].

To make full use of the superb PET-CT imaging, accurate target delineation becomes indispensable. Current standard medical practice heavily relies on manual contouring, which is performed visually on a slice-by-slice basis by radiation

M.J. Cardoso et al. (Eds.): CMMI/RAMBO/SWITCH 2017, LNCS 10555, pp. 31–42, 2017.
DOI: 10.1007/978-3-319-67564-0_4

oncologists for target delineation. Due to the nature of PET-CT imaging, manual contouring is cumbersome and error-prone, and suffers substantial inter- and intra-observer variability [4–7]. This may limit its use as a quantitative imaging tool or biomarker of outcome/response in large-scale clinical trial research and even for use in daily clinical care.

Substantial endeavors have been made on automated tumor definition from PET-CT scans using, for example, standardized uptake values (SUVs) based thresholding [8–11], image gradients [12,13], deformable contour models [14–16], mutual information in hybrid [17–19], random walk [20], and Gaussian mixture models for heterogeneous regions [21,22]. Recently, the co-segmentation technique for tumor delineation on both PET and CT images has been attracted great attentions [18,23–26], in which tumor contours on PET and on CT are segmented simultaneously while admitting their possible differences. As demonstrated in those previous works, the design of cost functions in the framework of graph based co-segmentation is critical to achieve good segmentation performance. Consequently, the region/unary costs were usually carefully designed based on some sophisticated image priors (e.g., Gaussian mixture models [18,23], shape prior [26], texture information [25], etc.) or clinical information from expertise [23–26], and often heavily rely on hyper-parameters selection (e.g., the number of models in Gaussian mixture models [18], the curvature parameters [26], etc.) for improved results.

In this paper, we propose a novel 3D alpha matting technique to compute the region costs for co-segmentation on PET-CT images. The "matte" values computed from the 3D matting are used to design the region costs in the co-segmentation model [23]. Compared to previous PET-CT segmentation approaches, the proposed method is completely image-derived with less image and clinical priors, and consequently with less hyper-parameters. By integrating the 3D alpha matting technique into the context-aware co-segmentation framework [23], the proposed PET-CT co-segmentation method eases the design of cost functions for segmentation, and significantly outperforms the state-of-the-art PET-CT segmentation approach [23]. Note that although 3D matting has been used as post-processing for the refinement of segmentation [27,28], no previous work has been done using it for cost function design in the segmentation framework based on graph algorithms.

2   Methodology

The proposed PET-CT tumor segmentation method is semi-automated, which mainly consists of three steps: (1) Active contour is adopted to generate larger seed regions from given initial seeds on PET and CT image pairs, respectively. (2) Based on the new seed regions, 3D image matting are conducted in both volumes to obtain the tumor object probability maps, which are further used for computing region/unary costs for the co-segmentation model [23]. (3) The co-segmentation in both PET and CT modalities is formulated as a context constrained energy minimization problem, as in Song *et al.*'s method [23], which

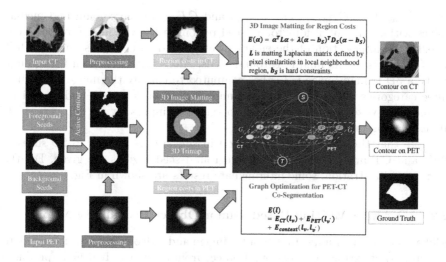

Fig. 1. The flowchart of proposed PET-CT co-segmentation framework.

can be solved optimally by the well-known max-flow/min-cut algorithm to obtain the simultaneous tumor segmentation result. The flowchart is shown in Fig. 1. In the following, we will describe those three steps in detail.

2.1 Active Contour Based 3D Trimap Generation

As a standard yet important procedure in medical image processing, a pre-processing step is needed in our framework. Similar to [23, 26], the PET images are first co-registered and up-sampled to have one-to-one voxel correspondence with the CT image. For each PET-CT image pair, initial foreground seeds (i.e., voxels that definitely belong to tumor object) and a background region (i.e., voxels that definitely do not belong to tumor object) are given with user interaction (for example, by drawing two spheres: the inner one indicates the tumor seeds and the region outside the outer sphere represents the background seeds). For CT image, we cut the intensity values (Hounsfield Units, HU) to the range of $[-500, 200]$ as possible tumor voxels to ignore irrelevant image details. For PET image, as suggested in literature, the raw image intensities are converted to standardized uptake values (SUV) according to de-identified patient meta-information.

Then, for each PET-CT pair, based on the given foreground seeds, the active contour technique is employed on the PET and CT images, respectively. As a consequence, we obtain an enlarged seed region on PET and CT images. However, due to the complex nature of a CT image, non-tumor voxels might also be included in the enlarged seed region, which would lead to inaccurate segmentation. To alleviate this problem, we remove some voxels by simply thresholding to keep those voxels whose HU values are in a specific range. The lower and upper bound of this range in HU are empirically set to $\max(-412, 0.1 * CT_{med})$ and

$\min(CT_{max}, 1.5 * CT_{med})$. The CT_{max} and CT_{med} are maximum and median values within the initial foreground seed region on the CT image, respectively. Finally, the intersection of the enlarged foreground seed regions on both PET and CT serves as the final foreground seeds. Along with the given background seeds, a 3D trimap image is further computed to classify the image voxels into three categories of regions (i.e., the tumor region, background, and the mixed or uncertain voxel region), which will be given as inputs for the subsequent 3D alpha matting procedure.

Note that the active contour method in this step is applied to 2D slices of PET and CT images where initial foreground seed regions are given. For the purpose of illustration, some intermediate results are shown in Fig. 1.

2.2 3D Alpha Matting Based Tumor Object Probability Maps

Alpha matting is an important tool for image and video editing, which refers to the process of extracting foreground object from an image. It usually produces a "matte" image that can be used to separate the foreground from the background in a given image. Suppose that an image I is composed of two parts: the foreground object F and the background B. The gray or color intensity of the i-th pixel is assumed to be a linear combination of the corresponding foreground (object) and background intensities: $I_i = \alpha_i \cdot F_i + (1 - \alpha_i) \cdot B_i$ where α_i, F_i and B_i are, respectively, the matte, the foreground, and the background (intensity) values of the i-th pixel. Alpha matting aims to simultaneously compute all three values for each pixel in one image by considering a "local smoothness assumption" that both F and B are approximately constant vector over a small local neighborhood window around each pixel. Inspired by the closed-form matting [29], we extend the 2D alpha matting to 3D and propose to adopt the "matte" values to compute tumor object probability maps used for region cost computation in the subsequent co-segmentation.

Specifically, given an image with a size of $H \times W \times D$, the local smoothness assumption allows us to reformulate the "alpha" for each voxel j in the 3D image I as $\alpha_j \approx a \cdot I_j + b, \forall j \in w$, where $a = \frac{1}{F_j - B_j}, b = -\frac{B_j}{F_j - B_j}$, w is a small neighborhood window. The goal of 3D alpha matting is to find the alpha for each voxel, which can be modeled as the following problem:

$$J(\alpha, a, b) = \sum_{j=1}^{N} \left[\sum_{i=1}^{|w_j|} (\alpha_j - a_j I_i - b_j)^2 + \epsilon a_j^2 \right] = \sum_{j=1}^{N} \left[\left\| \begin{bmatrix} I_1^j & 1 \\ I_2^j & 1 \\ \vdots & \vdots \\ I_{|w_j|}^j & 1 \\ \sqrt{\epsilon} & 0 \end{bmatrix} \begin{bmatrix} a_j \\ b_j \end{bmatrix} - \begin{bmatrix} \alpha_1^j \\ \alpha_2^j \\ \vdots \\ \alpha_{|w_j|}^j \\ 0 \end{bmatrix} \right\|^2 \right], \quad (1)$$

where $|w_j|$ is the number of voxel in j-th voxel neighborhood w_j, I_k^j and α_k^j ($k = \{1, \cdots, |w_j|\}$) are intensity and alpha values of k-th neighbor of j-th voxel, respectively. ϵ is a regularization constant. Using matrix notation, we have

$$J(\alpha, a, b) = \sum_{j=1}^{N} \left\| G_j \begin{bmatrix} a_j \\ b_j \end{bmatrix} - \bar{\alpha}_j \right\|^2. \tag{2}$$

Then, for each voxel j, we need to solve $a_j \in \mathbb{R}$, $b_j \in \mathbb{R}$ and $\bar{\alpha}_j \in \mathbb{R}^{(|w_j|+1)\times 1}$. Suppose we knew $\bar{\alpha}_j$, then we can obtain the optimal a_j and b_j as

$$\begin{bmatrix} a_j \\ b_j \end{bmatrix}^* = (G_j^T G_j)^{-1} G_j^T \bar{\alpha}_j, \tag{3}$$

then substituting this solution back into (2) and denoting $\bar{G}_j = I_{(|w_j|+1)\times(|w_j|+1)} - G_j (G_j^T G_j)^{-1} G_j^T \in \mathbb{R}^{(|w_j|+1)\times(|w_j|+1)}$, we obtain the α-subproblem as

$$J(\alpha) = \sum_{j=1}^{N} \left\| \bar{G}_j \bar{\alpha}_j \right\|^2 = \sum_{j=1}^{N} \bar{\alpha}_j^T \bar{G}_j^T \bar{G}_j \bar{\alpha}_j, \tag{4}$$

It is easily shown that $\bar{G}_j^T \bar{G}_j = I_{(|w_j|+1)\times(|w_j|+1)} - G_j (G_j^T G_j)^{-1} G_j^T$, $G_j^T G_j = \begin{bmatrix} \sum_{i=1}^{|w_j|} I_i^2 + \epsilon \sum_{i=1}^{|w_j|} I_i \\ \sum_{i=1}^{|w_j|} I_i & |w_j| \end{bmatrix}$ and $(G_j^T G_j)^{-1} = \frac{1}{|w_j|} \frac{1}{\left(\frac{\epsilon}{|w_j|}+\sigma_j^2\right)} \begin{bmatrix} 1 & -\mu_j \\ -\mu_j & \mu_j^2 + \sigma_j^2 + \frac{\epsilon}{|w_j|} \end{bmatrix}$, where μ_j and σ_j^2 are the mean and variance of the intensities in neighborhood window w_j (typically with a size of $3 \times 3 \times 3$) around j-th voxel, and $|w_j|$ is the number of voxels in the voxel set w_j. Finally, after some simple mathematical operations, the α-subproblem is formulated as

$$\alpha = \arg\min_{\alpha} \alpha^T L \alpha, \tag{5}$$

where $\alpha \in \mathbb{R}^{N \times 1}$ is the alpha matte vector for all $N = W \times H \times D$ voxels, and $L \in \mathbb{R}^{N \times N}$ is the matting Laplacian matrix, with (i, k)-entry being

$$\sum_{j|(i,k)\in w_j} \left(\delta_{ik} - \frac{1}{|w_j|} \left[1 + \frac{1}{\left(\frac{\epsilon}{|w_j|}+\sigma_j^2\right)} (I_i - \mu_j)(I_k - \mu_j) \right] \right), \tag{6}$$

where δ_{ik} is the Kronecker delta. However, the above problem (5) has singular solution. Thus, by considering user-supplied constraints on alpha values as in [29], the 3D alpha matting problem is finally formulated as:

$$\alpha = \arg\min_{\alpha} \alpha^T L \alpha + \lambda (\alpha^T - b_S^T) D_S (\alpha - b_S), \tag{7}$$

where λ is a coefficient, D_S is a diagonal matrix with an element 1 for each constrained voxel and with an element 0 for each of the remaining voxels, b_S is a vector indicating the alpha values for the constrained voxels. Since (7) is quadratic in alpha, we can obtain the final global optimum solution by solving a sparse linear system [29].

By considering the neighborhood relationships among spatially-adjacent and slice-adjacent voxels (e.g., w_j neighborhood for voxel j), the constructed matting Laplacian matrix L can better model tumor object structures, and consequently the probability generated from alpha matting would produce better segmentation results, which is validated in our experiments.

2.3 Context-Aware Co-segmentation

The context-aware graph cut based co-segmentation has been studied for tumor delineation on dual-modality PET-CT images [23]. Two sub-graphs are respectively constructed for both PET and CT images. Each sub-graph is constructed in a similar way as that in traditional graph cut based segmentation [30]. The edge weights in each sub-graph encode the region (or unary) and boundary (or pairwise) information from the corresponding image. In co-segmentation, a key ingredient lies in the incorporation of context information between the PET and CT images, which enforces the context-aware segmentation consistency between the corresponding nodes in the two sub-graphs by adding inter-edges between two sub-graphs. The co-segmentation is finally formulated as the following energy minimization problem that can be solved by the well-known maximum flow algorithm:

$$E\left(l\right) = E_{CT}\left(l\right) + \beta E_{PET}\left(l\right) + E_{context}\left(l\right) \tag{8}$$

$$E_{CT}\left(l\right) = \sum_{v \in \mathcal{I}} D_v\left(l_v\right) + \lambda_1 \sum_{(u,v) \in \mathcal{N}_{CT}} V_{uv}\left(l_u, l_v\right) \tag{9}$$

$$E_{PET}\left(l\right) = \sum_{v' \in \mathcal{I}'} D_{v'}\left(l_{v'}\right) + \lambda_2 \sum_{(u',v') \in \mathcal{N}_{PET}} V_{u'v'}\left(l_{u'}, l_{v'}\right) \tag{10}$$

$$E_{context}\left(l\right) = \sum_{(v,v')} W_{vv'}\left(l_v, l_{v'}\right) \tag{11}$$

where $\mathcal{I}$ denotes the input CT image, $\mathcal{I}'$ denotes the input co-registered PET image, l_v and $l_{v'}$ denote the binary labels assigned to each voxel $v \in \mathcal{I}$ and $v' \in \mathcal{I}'$, respectively. $D_v(l_v)$ and $V_{u,v}(l_u, l_v)$ denote the region and the boundary costs of each node (voxel) v on CT, respectively. $D_{v'}(l_{v'})$ and $V_{u'v'}(l_{u'}, l_{v'})$ denote the region, and the boundary costs of each node (voxel) v' on the PET image, respectively. $W_{vv'}(l_v, l_{v'})$ is a context-ware cost function. β, λ_1 and λ_2 are user-defined weight coefficients. $\mathcal{N}_{CT}$ and $\mathcal{N}_{PET}$ are the neighborhood systems defined on CT and PET, respectively.

In previous co-segmentation methods, $D_v(l_v)$ is often computed based on Gaussian mixture model [23] or integration of other complex image priors (e.g., shape prior [26]), while $D_{v'}(l_{v'})$ is usually specially-designed based on clinical information (e.g., empirically-thresholded SUV values [23,26], 3D derivative costs [26], etc.). In our work, an important difference is that those region costs are generated directly from the alpha mattes computed by the 3D image matting. Take as an example the voxel v in the CT image. The region terms take the form $D_v(l_v = 1) = -\log(\alpha_v)$ and $D_v(l_v = 0) = -\log(1 - \alpha_v)$ where α_v is the alpha matte value. For the design of the boundary term and the context term, we use a similar strategy as that in [23]. For the completeness, we summarize these terms here, as follows:

$$V_{uv}(l_u, l_v) = -\log\left(1 - \exp\left(\frac{-|\nabla\mathcal{I}|^2(u,v)}{2\sigma_{CT}^2}\right)\right) \qquad (12)$$

$$V_{u'v'}(l_{u'}, l_{v'}) = -\log\left(1 - \exp\left(\frac{-|\nabla\mathcal{I}'|^2(u',v')}{2\sigma_{PET}^2}\right)\right) \qquad (13)$$

$$W_{v,v'} = \theta\left(1 - |N_v - N_{v'}|\right) \qquad (14)$$

where $|\nabla\mathcal{I}|^2(u,v)$ denotes the squared gradient magnitude on CT between u and v. σ_{CT} and σ_{PET} are Gaussian kernel parameters. N_v and $N_{v'}$ are alpha mattes between $[0,1]$ obtained from the CT and PET images, respectively. θ is a scaling parameter.

3   Experiment

3.1   Datasets

A total of 54 PET-CT scan pairs from different patients with primary non-small cell lung cancer are obtained. The image spacing varies from $0.78 \times 0.78 \times 2\,\text{mm}^3$ to $1.27 \times 1.27 \times 3.4\,\text{mm}^3$. The intra slice image size is 512×512. The number of slices varies from 112 to 293. Manual expert tracings of the primary tumor volume is available for each scan.

The 54 scans are separated disjointly as a 10-scan training set and 44-scan testing set. The selection procedure starts by sorting all scans according to tumor volume. Then one scan out of every five scan is selected as training scan. This stratified strategy makes sure the training set is representative of the whole population in terms of tumor volume. All parameters are tuned on the training set. All reported results are from the testing set.

3.2   Experiment Settings

The same initialization procedure in [23] is employed. The user first specify two concentric spheres with the different radii to serve as object and background seeds. More specifically, all voxels inside the smaller sphere are used as object seed. All voxels outside the larger sphere are used as background seed.

The segmentation accuracy is measured by the Dice coefficient (DSC). Dice coefficient measures the volume overlap of two segmentations A and B. It is defined as $2|A \cap B|/(|A| + |B|)$, with a range of $[0,1]$. The higher the DSC is, the better volume overlap the two segmentations have.

A grid search strategy is used to select the parameters. The parameters returning highest training set DSC is used to run the co-segmentation on the test set. The values of those parameters are set, as follows: $\beta = 5$, $\lambda_1 = 5$, $\lambda_2 = 0.1$, $\sigma_{CT} = 15$, $\sigma_{PET} = 0.1$, and $\theta = 255$.

We conducted quantitative comparisons to the state-of-the-art PET-CT co-segmentation method of Song et al.'s [23]. For better illustration of the alpha-mattes based region costs for (co-)segmentation, two groups of experiments were conducted. In the first group, the context term was not used, and the traditional graph cut based segmentation method [30] was applied solely on CT or PET for tumor segmentation using our proposed mattes based cost functions. In the second group of experiments, both PET and CT scans were used for our co-segmentation of tumor contours.

3.3   Results and Analysis

Table 1 reports the mean DSCs and standard deviations of the evaluated methods on the 44 test datasets. Figure 2 shows their quantitative results for each method on each case. From these results, we have the following observations. First, compared to Song's co-segmentation method, our matte based method can achieve better performance on most cases with higher DSCs (on average, 3.4% improvement) with a significant confidence (p-value of 0.005). Second, from the results of either Song's or our method, the co-segmentation can achieve better results over the traditional graph cut segmentation methods (i.e., the superiority of co-Seg. over CT-only or PET-only). Third, considering the traditional graph cut based segmentation (i.e., without context-aware information between inter-

Table 1. Average DSC's and standard deviations of the proposed method and Song et al.'s co-segmentation method [23].

Methods	Modalities	DSC	p-values
Song et al. [23]	CT-only	0.495 ± 0.208	
	PET-only	0.582 ± 0.134	
	PET-CT	0.768 ± 0.114	
Proposed	CT-only	0.744 ± 0.101	10^{-10}
	PET-only	0.757 ± 0.077	10^{-13}
	PET-CT	0.802 ± 0.069	0.005

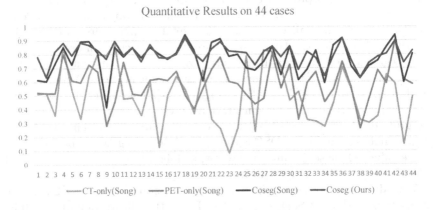

Fig. 2. Quantitative results and comparative performance evaluation based on the computed DSC values.

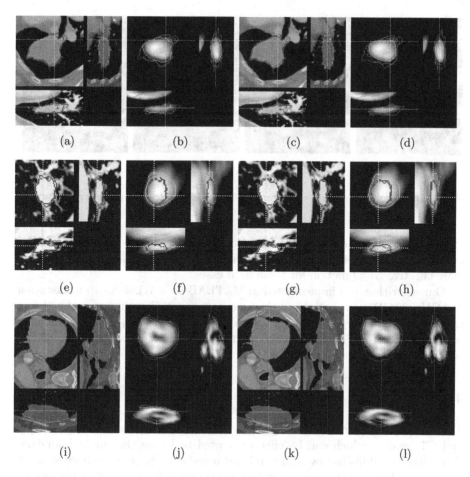

Fig. 3. Segmentation results of compared methods on three PET-CT scans: No. 000577, 001255 and 001263 (from the first row to the last row). The 1st and 2nd columns: contours on CT and PET images *with* co-segmentation. The 3rd and 4th columns: contours on CT and PET images *without* co-segmentation. Red: ground truth, Green: Song's method, Blue: Our method. (Color figure online)

subgraphs), the segmentation results using the proposed region costs generated by 3D alpha matting outperformed those using Song *et al.*'s region costs.

Qualitatively, Fig. 3 shows the segmentation results of the compared methods on three PET-CT scans. From those figures, we can see our method is able to locate tumor boundary more accurately. Note that the ground truth was only given on CT images, we draw the contours on PET images for demonstration.

It is noted that although our method can achieve good segmentation results on most cases, it still cannot handle some hard cases. One example case for which our method achieved less accurate segmentation is shown in Fig. 4. As we can see in this figure, although our method can localize the obvious tumor boundary

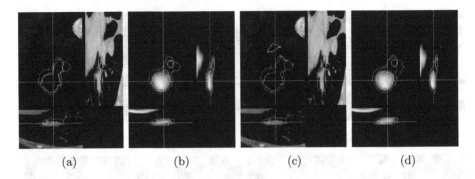

(a)   (b)   (c)   (d)

Fig. 4. One example case for which our method achieved less accurate segmentation.

on CT images, it is difficult to recognize those voxels with extremely low HU values in tumor region. Possible improvements in the future lies in how to design more effective cost function for these hard cases.

Our algorithm was implemented in MATLAB on a Windows 10 workstation (3.4 GHz, 32 GB memory). As to the average computation time over the 44 test cases, the 3D image matting step took about 43.49 s, the co-segmentation step took about 68.76 s. Thus, our method took about 2 min for each case, which was comparable to those reported in [23].

4   Conclusion

The novel 3D image matting can generate high-quality region cost on both PET and CT images, which can be effectively used to locate the tumor boundary. When integrated in the powerful graph cut based co-segmentation framework, it can achieve high accurate segmentation for tumor delineation. Experiments on 54 datasets demonstrated the effectiveness of the proposed method.

Acknowledgments. This research was supported in part by the NIH Grant R21CA209874.

References

1. Hatt, M., Tixier, F., Pierce, L., Kinahan, P., Le Rest, C., Visvikis, D.: Characterization of PET/CT images using texture analysis: the past, the present... any future? Eur. J. Nucl. Med. Mol. Imaging **44**(1), 151–166 (2017)
2. Bagci, U., Udupa, J.K., Mendhiratta, N., Foster, B., Xu, Z., Yao, J., Chen, X., Mollura, D.J.: Joint segmentation of anatomical and functional images: applications in quantification of lesions from PET, PET-CT, MRI-PET, and MRI-PET-CT images. Med. Image Anal. **17**(8), 929–945 (2013)
3. Foster, B., Bagci, U., Mansoor, A., Xu, Z., Mollura, D.J.: A review on segmentation of positron emission tomography images. Comput. Biol. Med. **50**, 76–96 (2014)

4. Steenbakkers, R.J.H.M., Duppen, J.C., Fitton, I., Deurloo, K.E.I., Zijp, L.J., Comans, E.F.I., Uitterhoeve, A.L.J., Rodrigus, P.T.R., Kramer, G.W.P., Bussink, J., De Jaeger, K., Belderbos, J.S.A., Nowak, P.J.C.M., van Herk, M., Rasch, C.R.N.: Reduction of observer variation using matched CT-PET for lung cancer delineation: a threee-dimensional analysis. Int. J. Radiat. Oncol. Biol. Phys. **64**, 435–448 (2006)

5. Fiorino, C., Reni, M., Bolognesi, A., Cattaneo, G., Calandrino, R.: Intra- and inter-observer variability in contouring prostate and seminal vesicles: implications for conformal treatment planning. Int. J. Radiat. Oncol. Biol. Phys. **4**, 285–292 (1998)

6. Chang, J., Joon, D.L., Lee, S., Gong, S., Anderson, N., Scott, A., Davis, I., Clouston, D., Bolton, D., Hamilton, C., Khoo, V.: Intensity modulated radiation therapy dose painting for localized prostate cancer using ^{11}C-choline positron emission tomography scans. Int. J. Radiat. Oncol. Biol. Phys. **83**(5), 691–696 (2012)

7. Breen, S.L., Publicover, J., De Silva, S., Pond, G., Brock, K., OSullivan, B., Cummings, B., Dawson, L., Keller, A., Kim, J., Ringash, J., Yu, E., Hendler, A., Waldron, J.: Intraobserver and interobserver variability in GTV delineation on FDG-PET-CT images of head and neck cancers. Int. J. Radiat. Oncol. Biol. Phys. **68**, 763–770 (2007)

8. Hong, R., Halama, J., Bova, D., Sethi, A., Emami, B.: Correlation of PET standard uptake value and CT window-level thresholds for target delineation in CT-based radiation treatment planning. Int. J. Radiat. Oncol. Biol. Phys. **67**, 720–726 (2007)

9. Erdi, Y.E., Mawlawi, O., Larson, S.M., Imbriaco, M., Yeung, H., Finn, R., Humm, J.L.: Segmentation of lung lesion volume by adaptive positron emission tomography image thresholding. Cancer **80**, 2505–2509 (1997)

10. Miller, T.R., Grigsby, P.W.: Measurement of tumor volume by PET to evaluate prognosis in patients with advanced cervical cancer treated by radiation therapy. Int. J. Radiat. Oncol. Biol. Phys. **53**, 353–359 (2002)

11. Nehmeh, S.A., El-Zeftawy, H., Greco, C., Schwartz, J., Erdi, Y.E., Kirov, A., Schmidtlein, C.R., Gyau, A.B., Larson, S.M., Humm, J.L.: An iterative technique to segment PET lesions using a Monte Carlo based mathematical model. Med. Phys. **36**, 4803–4809 (2009)

12. Drever, L., Roa, W., McEwan, A., Robinson, D.: Comparison of three image segmentation techniques for target volume delineation in positron emission tomography. J. Appl. Clin. Med. Phys. **8**, 93–109 (2007)

13. Geets, X., Lee, J., Bol, A., Lonneux, M., Gregoire, V.: A gradient-based method for segmenting FDG-PET images: methodology and validation. Eur. J. Nucl. Med. Mol. Imaging **34**, 1427–1438 (2007)

14. Hsu, C.Y., Liu, C.Y., Chen, C.M.: Automatic segmentation of liver PET images. Med. Phys. **32**, 601–610 (2008)

15. Li, H., Thorstad, W.L., Biehl, K.J., Laforest, R., Su, Y., Shoghi, K.I., Donnelly, E.D., Low, D.A., Lu, W.: A novel PET tumor delineation method based on adaptive region-growing and dual-front active contours. Med. Phys. **35**, 3711–3721 (2008)

16. El Naqa, I., Yang, D., Apte, A., Khullar, D., Mutic, S., Zheng, J., Bradley, J.D., Grigsby, P., Deasy, J.O.: Concurrent multimodality image segmentation by active contours for radiotherapy treatment planning. Med. Phys. **34**(12), 4738–4749 (2007)

17. Grubben, H., Miller, P., Hanna, G., Carson, K., Hounsell, A.: MAP-MRF segmentation of lung tumours in PET-CT image. In: Proceedings of International Symposium on Biomedical Imaging, pp. 290–293 (2009)

18. Han, D., Bayouth, J., Song, Q., Taurani, A., Sonka, M., Buatti, J., Wu, X.: Globally optimal tumor segmentation in PET-CT images: a graph-based co-segmentation method. In: Székely, G., Hahn, H.K. (eds.) IPMI 2011. LNCS, vol. 6801, pp. 245–256. Springer, Heidelberg (2011). doi:10.1007/978-3-642-22092-0_21

19. Aristophanous, M., Penney, B., Martel, M., Pelizzari, C.: A gaussian mixture model for definition of lung tumor volumes in positron emission tomography. Med. Phys. **34**, 4223–4235 (2007)

20. Bagci, U., Udupa, J.K., Yao, J., Mollura, D.J.: Co-segmentation of functional and anatomical images. In: Ayache, N., Delingette, H., Golland, P., Mori, K. (eds.) MICCAI 2012. LNCS, vol. 7512, pp. 459–467. Springer, Heidelberg (2012). doi:10.1007/978-3-642-33454-2_57

21. Foster, B., Bagci, U., Luna, B., Dey, B., Bishai, W., Jain, S., Xu, Z., Mollura, D.: Robust segmentation and accurate target definition for positron emission tomography images using affinity propagation. In: 2013 IEEE 10th International Symposium on Biomedical Imaging (ISBI), pp. 1461–1464, April 2013

22. Hatt, M., le Rest, C.C., Turzo, A., Roux, C., Visvikis, D.: A fuzzy locally adaptive Bayesian segmentation approach for volume determination in PET. IEEE Trans. Med. Imaging **28**, 881–893 (2009)

23. Song, Q., Bai, J., Han, D., Bhatia, S., Sun, W., Rockey, W., Bayouth, J.E., Buatti, J.M., Wu, X.: Optimal co-segmentation of tumor in PET-CT images with context information. IEEE Trans. Med. Imaging **32**(9), 1685–1697 (2013)

24. Li, H., Bai, J., Hejle, T.A., Wu, X., Bhatia, S., Kim, Y.: Automated cosegmentation of tumor volume and metabolic activity using PET-CT in non-small cell lung cancer (NSCLC). Int. J. Radiat. Oncol. Biol. Phys. **87**(2), S528 (2013)

25. Lartizien, C., Rogez, M., Niaf, E., Ricard, F.: Computer-aided staging of lymphoma patients with FDG PET/CT imaging based on textural information. IEEE J. Biomed. Health Inf. **18**(3), 946–955 (2014)

26. Ju, W., Xiang, D., Zhang, B., Wang, L., Kopriva, I., Chen, X.: Random walk and graph cut for co-segmentation of lung tumor on PET-CT images. IEEE Trans. Image Process. **24**(12), 5854–5867 (2015)

27. Shao, H.C., Cheng, W.Y., Chen, Y.C., Hwang, W.L.: Colored multi-neuron image processing for segmenting and tracing neural circuits. In: 2012 19th IEEE International Conference on Image Processing, pp. 2025–2028, September 2012

28. Zeng, Z., Zwiggelaar, R.: Segmentation for multiple sclerosis lesions based on 3D volume enhancement and 3D alpha matting. In: Kamel, M., Campilho, A. (eds.) ICIAR 2013. LNCS, vol. 7950, pp. 573–580. Springer, Heidelberg (2013). doi:10.1007/978-3-642-39094-4_65

29. Levin, A., Lischinski, D., Weiss, Y.: A closed-form solution to natural image matting. IEEE Trans. Pattern Anal. Mach. Intell. **30**(2), 228–242 (2008)

30. Boykov, Y., Funka-Lea, G.: Graph cuts and efficient N-D image segmentation. Int. J. Comput. Vis. **70**(2), 109–131 (2006)

Synthesis of Positron Emission Tomography (PET) Images via Multi-channel Generative Adversarial Networks (GANs)

Lei Bi[1]([✉]), Jinman Kim[1], Ashnil Kumar[1], Dagan Feng[1,2],
and Michael Fulham[1,3,4]

[1] School of Information Technologies, University of Sydney, Sydney, Australia
lei.bi@sydney.edu.au
[2] Med-X Research Institute, Shanghai Jiao Tong University, Shanghai, China
[3] Department of Molecular Imaging, Royal Prince Alfred Hospital,
Sydney, Australia
[4] Sydney Medical School, University of Sydney, Sydney, Australia

Abstract. Positron emission tomography (PET) imaging is widely used for staging and monitoring treatment in a variety of cancers including the lymphomas and lung cancer. Recently, there has been a marked increase in the accuracy and robustness of machine learning methods and their application to computer-aided diagnosis (CAD) systems, e.g., the automated detection and quantification of abnormalities in medical images. Successful machine learning methods require large amounts of training data and hence, synthesis of PET images could play an important role in enhancing training data and ultimately improve the accuracy of PET-based CAD systems. Existing approaches such as atlas-based or methods that are based on simulated or physical phantoms have problems in synthesizing the low resolution and low signal-to-noise ratios inherent in PET images. In addition, these methods usually have limited capacity to produce a variety of synthetic PET images with large anatomical and functional differences. Hence, we propose a new method to synthesize PET data via multi-channel generative adversarial networks (M-GAN) to address these limitations. Our M-GAN approach, in contrast to the existing medical image synthetic methods that rely on using low-level features, has the ability to capture feature representations with a high-level of semantic information based on the adversarial learning concept. Our M-GAN is also able to take the input from the annotation (label) to synthesize regions of high uptake e.g., tumors and from the computed tomography (CT) images to constrain the appearance consistency based on the CT derived anatomical information in a single framework and output the synthetic PET images directly. Our experimental data from 50 lung cancer PET-CT studies show that our method provides more realistic PET images compared to conventional GAN methods. Further, the PET tumor detection model, trained with our synthetic PET data, performed competitively when compared to the detection model trained with real PET data (2.79% lower in terms of recall). We suggest that our approach when used in combination with real and synthetic images, boosts the training data for machine learning methods.

© Springer International Publishing AG 2017
M.J. Cardoso et al. (Eds.): CMMI/RAMBO/SWITCH 2017, LNCS 10555, pp. 43–51, 2017.
DOI: 10.1007/978-3-319-67564-0_5

Keywords: Positron Emission Tomography (PET) · Generative Adversarial Networks (GANs) · Image synthesis

1 Introduction

[18F]-Fluorodeoxyglucose (FDG) positron emission tomography (PET) is widely used for staging, and monitoring the response to treatment in a wide variety of cancers, including the lymphoma and lung cancer [1–3]. This is attributed to the ability of FDG PET to depict regions of increased glucose metabolism in sites of active tumor relative to normal tissues [1,4]. Recently, advances in machine learning methods have been applied to medical computer-aided diagnosis (CAD) [5], where algorithms such as deep learning and pattern recognition, can provide automated detection of abnormalities in medical images [6–8]. Machine learning methods are dependent on the availability of large amounts of annotated data for training and for the derivation of learned models [7,8]. There is, however, a scarcity of annotated training data for medical images which relates to the time involved in manual annotation and the confirmation of the imaging findings [9,10]. Further, the training data need to encompass the wide variation in the imaging findings of a particular disease across a number of different patients. Hence effort has been directed in deriving other sources of training data such as 'synthetic' images. Early approaches used simulated, e.g., Monte Carlo approaches [24,25] or physical phantoms that consisted of simplified anatomical structures [11]. Unfortunately, phantoms are unable to generate high-quality synthetic images and cannot simulate a wide variety of complex interactions, e.g., presence of the deformations introduced by disease. Other investigators used atlases [12] where different transformation maps were applied on the atlas with an intensity fusion technique to create new images. However, atlas based methods usually require many pre-/post-processing steps and a priori knowledge for tuning large amounts of transformation parameters, and thus limiting their ability to be widely adopted. Further, image registration that is used for creating the transformation maps affects the quality of the synthetic images.

In this paper, we propose a new method to produce synthetic PET images using a multi-channel generative adversarial network (M-GAN). Our method exploits the state-of-the-art GAN image synthesis approach [13–16] with a novel adaptation for PET images and key improvements. The success of GAN is based on its ability to capture feature representations that contain a high-level of semantic information using the adversarial learning concept. A GAN has two competing neural networks, where the first neural network is trained to find an optimal mapping between the input data to the synthetic images, while the second neural network is trained to detect the generated synthetic images from the real images. Therefore, the optimal feature representation is acquired during the adversarial learning process. Although GANs have had great success in the generation of natural images, its application to PET images is not trivial. There are three main ways to conduct PET image synthesis with GAN: (1) PET-to-PET; (2) Label-to-PET; and (3) Computed tomography (CT)-to-PET.

For PET-to-PET synthesis, it is challenging to create new variations of the input PET images, since the mapping from the input to the synthetic PET cannot be markedly different. Label-to-PET synthesis usually has limited constraints in synthesizing PET images, so the synthesized PET images can lack spatial and appearance consistency, e.g., the lung tumor appears outside the thorax. CT-to-PET synthesis is not usually able to synthesize high uptake regions e.g., tumors, since the high uptake regions may not be always visible as an abnormality on the CT images. Both PET-to-PET and CT-to-PET synthesis require new annotations for the new synthesized PET images for machine learning. Our proposition to address these limitations is a multi-channel GAN where we take the annotations (labels) to synthesize the high uptake regions and then the corresponding CT images to constrain the appearance consistency and output the synthetic PET images. The label is not necessary to be derived from the corresponding CT image, where user can draw any high uptake regions on the CT images which are going to be synthesized. The novelty of our method, compared to prior approaches, is as follows: (1) it harnesses high-level semantic information for effective PET image synthesis in an end-to-end manner that does not require pre-/post-processing or parameter tuning; (2) we propose a new multi-channel generative adversarial networks (M-GAN) for PET image synthesis. During training, M-GAN is capable of learning the integration from both CT and label to synthesize the high uptake and the anatomical background. During predication, M-GAN uses the label and the estimated synthetic PET images derived from CT to gradually improve the quality of the synthetic PET image; and (3) our synthetic PET images can be used to boost the training data for machine learning methods.

2 Methods

2.1 Multi-channel Generative Adversarial Networks (M-GANs)

GANs [13] have 2 main components: a generative model G (the generator) that captures the data distribution and a discriminative model D (the discriminator) that estimates the probability of a sample that came from the training data rather than G. The generator is trained to produce outputs that cannot be distinguished from the real data by the adversarially trained discriminator, while the discriminator was trained to detect the synthetic data created by the generator.

Therefore, the overall objective is to minimize min-max loss function, which is defined as:

$$L(G, D) = \mathbb{E}_{x \sim p_{data(x)}}[log D(x)] + \mathbb{E}_{z \sim p_{z(z)}}[log(1 - D(G(z)))] \qquad (1)$$

where x is the real data and z is the input random noise. p_{data}, p_z represent the distribution of the real data and the input noise. $D(x)$ represents the probability that x came from the real data while $G(z)$ represents the mapping to synthesize the real data.

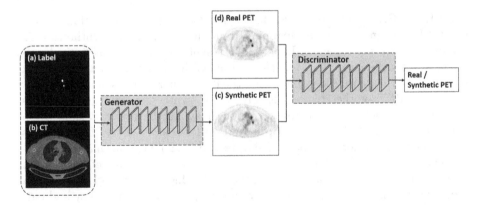

Fig. 1. Flow diagram of our M-GANs.

For our M-GAN, we embed the label and the CT image for training and testing, as shown in Fig. 1. During the training time, the generator takes input from the label and CT to learn a mapping to synthesize the real PET images. Then the synthesized PET images, together with the real PET images, enter into the discriminator for separation as:

$$L_{M-GAN}(G, D) = \mathbb{E}_{l,c,t\sim p_{data(l,c,t)}}[logD(l,c,t)] +$$
$$\mathbb{E}_{c\sim p_{c(c)},l\sim p_{l(l)}}[log(1 - D(l,c,G(l,c)))] \quad (2)$$

where l is the label, c the CT and t is the PET image. The conceptual approach to train the M-GAN is to find an optimal setting G^* that maximizes D while minimizing G, which can be defined as:

$$G^* = arg \min_G \max_D L_{M-GAN}(G, D) \quad (3)$$

Based on the latest empirical data reported by van den Oord et al. [14], we used $L1$ distance to encourage less blurring for the synthetic images during training. Therefore, the optimization process becomes:

$$G^* = arg \min_G \max_D L_{M-GAN}(G, D) + \lambda \mathbb{E}_{c\sim p_{c(c)},l\sim p_{l(l)}}[\|t - G(l,c)\|_1] \quad (4)$$

where λ is a hyper-parameter, which balances the contribution of the two terms and we set it to 100 empirically. We followed the published work Isola et al. [15] and used a U-net [17] architecture for the generator G and a five-layer convolutional networks for the discriminator D.

2.2   Materials and Implementation Details

Our dataset consisted of 50 PET-CT studies from 50 lung cancer patients provided by the Department of Molecular Imaging, Royal Prince Alfred (RPA) Hospital, Sydney, NSW, Australia. All studies were acquired on a 128-slice Siemens

Biograph mCT scanner; each study had a CT volume and a PET volume. The reconstructed volumes had a PET resolution of 200×200 pixels at $4.07\,\text{mm}^2$, CT resolution of 512×512 pixels at $0.98\,\text{mm}^2$ and slice thickness of $3\,\text{mm}$. All data were de-identified. Each study contained between 1 to 7 tumors. Tumors were initially detected with a 40% peak SUV (standardized uptake value) connected thresholding to detect 'hot spots'. We used the findings from the clinical reports to make manual adjustments to ensure that the segmented tumors were accurate. The reports provided the location of the tumors and any involved lymph nodes in the thorax. All scans were read by an experienced clinician who has read 60,000 PET-CT studies.

To evaluate our approach we carried out experiments only on trans-axial slices that contained tumors and so analyzed 876 PET-CT slices from 50 patient studies. We randomly separated these slices into two groups, each containing 25 patient studies. We used the first group as the training and tested on the second group, and then reversed the roles of the groups. We ensured that no patient PET-CT slices were in both training and test groups. Our method took 6 h to train over 200 epochs with a 12GB Maxwell Titan X GPU on the Torch library [18].

3 Evaluation

3.1 Experimental Results for PET Image Synthesis

We compared our M-GAN to single channel variants: the LB-GAN (using labels) and the CT-GAN (using CTs). We used mean absolute error (MAE) and peak signal-to-noise ratio (PSNR) for evaluating the different methods [19]. MAE measures the average distance between each corresponding pixels of the synthetic and the real PET image. PSNR measures the ratio between the maximum possible intensity value and the mean squared error of the synthetic and the real PET image. The results are shown in Table 1 where the M-GAN had the best performance across all measurements with the lowest MAE and highest PSNR.

Table 1. Comparison of the different GAN approaches.

	MAE	PSNR
LB-GAN	7.98	24.25
CT-GAN	4.77	26.65
M-GAN	**4.60**	**28.06**

3.2 Using Synthetic PET Images for Training

In the second experiment, we analysed the synthetic PET images to determine their contribution to train a fully convolutional network (FCN - a widely used

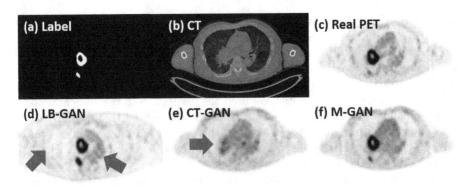

Fig. 2. Synthetic PET images. (a) label, (b) CT image, (c) real PET image, (d, e) synthetic PET images produced with only using (a) or (b), (f) our synthetic PET images with both (a) and (b) as the input.

deep convolutional networks for object detection task [20–22]). We trained the FCN model with (i) LB-GAN, (ii) CT-GAN, (iii) M-GAN produced synthetic or (iv) real PET images. Then we applied the trained FCN model to detect tumors on real PET images (We used the first group to build the GAN model and the GAN model was applied on the second group to produce the synthetic PET images. After that, the synthetic PET images were used to build the FCN model. Finally the trained FCN model was tested on the first group with the real PET images for tumor detection. We reversed the roles of the two groups and applied the same procedures). Our evaluation was based on the overlap ratio between the detected tumor and the ground truth annotations [23]. A detected tumor with >50% overlap with the annotated tumor (ground truth) was considered as true positive; additional detected tumor was considered as false positive. We regarded an annotated tumor that was not detected, or an overlap, smaller than 50%, between the detected tumor and the annotated tumors as false negative. We measured the overall precision, recall and f-score.

Table 2 shows the detection and segmentation performances. The results indicate that the M-GAN synthesized PET images performed competitively to the results produced from using real PET images for tumor detection.

Table 2. Comparision of FCN-based tumor detection performance, trained using synthetic or real PET.

Trained FCN with	Precision	Recall	F-score
LB-GAN PET	76.42	44.06	55.90
CT-GAN PET	36.89	3.69	6.71
M-GAN PET	81.73	52.38	63.84
Real PET	88.31	55.17	66.38

4   Discussion

Table 1 indicates that the M-GAN is much closer to the real images when compared with other GAN variants, and achieved the lowest MAE score of 4.60 and a highest PSNR of 28.06. The best score in both MAE and PSNR can be used to indicate the construction of the most useful synthetic images. In general, LB-GAN may be employed to boost the training data. However, due to the lack of spatial and appearance constraints that could be derived from CT, LB-GAN usually result in poor anatomical definitions, as exemplified in Fig. 2d, where the lung boundaries were missing and the mediastinum regions were synthesized wrongly.

CT-GAN achieved competitive results in terms of MAE and PSNR (Table 1). However, its limitation is with its inability to reconstruct the lesions which are information that is only available in the label images (or PET), as exemplified in Fig. 2e, where the two tumors were missing and one additional tumor was randomly appeared in the heart region from the synthetic images. The relative small differences between the proposed M-GAN method and CT-GAN method was due to the fact that tumor regions only occupy a small portion of the whole image and therefore, resulting less emphasis for the overall evaluation. In general, CT-GAN cannot synthesize the high uptake tumor regions, especially for the tumors adjacent to the mediastinum. This is further evidence in Table 2; CT-GAN synthesized PET images have inconsistent labeling of the tumors and resulting the trained FCN producing the lowest detection results.

In Table 2, the difference between the M-GAN and the detection results by using the real PET images demonstrate the advantages in integrating label to synthesize the tumors and the CT to constrain the appearance consistency in a single framework for training.

5   Conclusion

We propose a new M-GAN framework for synthesizing PET images by embedding a multi-channel input in a generative adversarial network and thereby enabling the learning of PET high uptake regions such as tumors and the spatial and appearance constraint from the CT data. Our preliminary results on 50 lung cancer PET-CT studies demonstrate that our method was much closer to the real PET images when compared to the conventional GAN approaches. More importantly, the PET tumor detection model trained with our synthetic PET images performed competitively to the same model trained with real PET images. In this work, we only evaluated the use of synthetic images to replace the original PET; in our future work, we will investigate novel approaches to optimally combine the real and synthetic images to boost the training data. We suggest that our framework can potentially boost the training data for machine learning algorithms that depends on large PET-CT data collection, and can also be extended to support other multi-modal data sets as PET-MRI synthesis.

References

1. Nestle, U., et al.: Comparison of different methods for delineation of 18F-FDG PET-positive tissue for target volume definition in radiotherapy of patients with non-small cell lung cancer. J. Nuclear Med. **46**, 1342–1348 (2005)
2. Li, H., et al.: A novel PET tumor delineation method based on adaptive region-growing and dual-front active contours. Med. Phys. **35**(8), 3711–3721 (2008)
3. Hoh, C.K., et al.: Whole-body FDG-PET imaging for staging of Hodgkin's disease and lymphoma. J. Nuclear Med. **38**(3), 343 (1997)
4. Bi, L., et al.: Automatic detection and classification of regions of FDG uptake in whole-body PET-CT lymphoma studies. Comput. Med. Imaging Graph. (2016). http://dx.doi.org/10.1016/j.compmedimag.2016.11.008. ISSN 0895-6111
5. Doi, K.: Computer-aided diagnosis in medical imaging: historical review, current status and future potential. Comput. Med. Imaging Graph. **31**(4), 198–211 (2007)
6. Gulshan, V., et al.: Development and validation of a deep learning algorithm for detection of diabetic retinopathy in retinal fundus photographs. JAMA **316**, 2402–2410 (2016)
7. Kooi, T., et al.: Large scale deep learning for computer aided detection of mammographic lesions. Med. Image Anal. **35**, 303–312 (2017)
8. Esteva, A., et al.: Dermatologist-level classification of skin cancer with deep neural networks. Nature **542**(7639), 115–118 (2017)
9. Chen, H., et al.: DCAN: Deep contour-aware networks for object instance segmentation from histology images. Med. Image Anal. **36**, 135–146 (2017)
10. Bi, L., et al.: Dermoscopic image segmentation via multi-stage fully convolutional networks. IEEE Trans. Biomed. Eng. **64**, 2065–2074 (2017)
11. Mumcuoglu, E.U., et al.: Bayesian reconstruction of PET images: methodology and performance analysis. Phys. Med. Biol. **41**, 1777 (1996)
12. Burgos, N., et al.: Attenuation correction synthesis for hybrid PET-MR scanners: application to brain studies. IEEE Trans. Med. Imaging **12**, 2332–2341 (2014)
13. Goodfellow, I., et al.: Generative adversarial nets. In: Neural Information Processing Systems (2014)
14. van den Oord, A., et al.: Conditional image generation with pixelcnn decoders. In: Neural Information Processing Systems (2016)
15. Isola, P., et al.: Image-to-image translation with conditional adversarial networks. In: Computer Vision and Pattern Recognition (2017)
16. Shrivastava, A., et al.: Learning from simulated and unsupervised images through adversarial training. arXiv preprint arXiv:1612.07828 (2016)
17. Ronneberger, O., Fischer, P., Brox, T.: U-Net: convolutional networks for biomedical image segmentation. In: Navab, N., Hornegger, J., Wells, W.M., Frangi, A.F. (eds.) MICCAI 2015. LNCS, vol. 9351, pp. 234–241. Springer, Cham (2015). doi:10.1007/978-3-319-24574-4_28
18. Collobert, R., Bengio, S., Mariéthoz, J.: Torch: a modular machine learning software library. No. EPFL-REPORT-82802. Idiap (2002)
19. Gholipour, A., et al.: Robust super-resolution volume reconstruction from slice acquisitions: application to fetal brain MRI. IEEE Trans. Med. Imaging **29**(10), 1739–1758 (2010)
20. Long, J., Shelhamer, E., Darrell, T.: Fully convolutional networks for semantic segmentation. In: Computer Vision and Pattern Recognition (2015)
21. Bi, L., et al.: Stacked fully convolutional networks with multi-channel learning: application to medical image segmentation. Vis. Comput. **33**(6), 1061–1071 (2017)

22. Kamnitsas, K., et al.: Efficient multi-scale 3D CNN with fully connected CRF for accurate brain lesion segmentation. Med. Image Anal. **36**, 61–78 (2017)
23. Song, Y., et al.: A multistage discriminative model for tumor and lymph node detection in thoracic images. IEEE Trans. Med. Imaging **31**(5), 1061–1075 (2012)
24. Kim, J., et al.: Use of anatomical priors in the segmentation of PET lung tumor images. In: Nuclear Science Symposium Conference Record, vol. 6, pp. 4242–4245 (2007)
25. Papadimitroulas, P., et al.: Investigation of realistic PET simulations incorporating tumor patient's specificity using anthropomorphic models: creation of an oncology database. Med. Phys. 40(11), 112506-(1-13) (2013)

Second International Workshop on Reconstruction and Analysis of Moving Body Organs, RAMBO 2017

Dynamic Respiratory Motion Estimation Using Patch-Based Kernel-PCA Priors for Lung Cancer Radiotherapy

Tiancheng He, Ramiro Pino, Bin Teh, Stephen Wong, and Zhong Xue[(⊠)]

Houston Methodist Research Institute, Weill Cornell Medicine, Houston, TX, USA
zxue@houstonmethodist.org

Abstract. In traditional radiation therapy of lung cancer, the planned target volume (PTV) is delineated from the average or a single phase of the planning-4D-CT, which is then registered to the intra-procedural 3D-CT for delivery of radiation dose. Because of respiratory motion, the radiation needs to be gated so that the PTV covers the tumor. 4D planning deals with multiple breathing phases, however, since the breathing patterns during treatment can change, there are matching discrepancies between the planned 4D volumes and the actual tumor shape and position. Recent works showed that it is promising to dynamically estimate the lung motion from chest motion. In this paper, we propose a patch-based Kernel-PCA model for estimating lung motion from the chest and upper abdomen motion. First, a statistical model is established from the 4D motion fields of a population. Then, the lung motion of a patient is estimated dynamically based on the patient's 4D-CT image and chest and upper abdomen motion, using population's statistical model as prior knowledge. This lung motion estimation algorithm aims to adapt the patient's planning 4D-CT to his/her current breathing status dynamically during treatment so that the location and shape of the lung tumor can be precisely tracked. Thus, it reduces possible damage to surrounding normal tissue, reduces side-effects, and improves the efficiency of radiation therapy. In experiments, we used the leave-one-out method to evaluate the estimation accuracy from images of 51 male subjects and compared the linear and nonlinear estimation scenarios. The results showed smaller lung field matching errors for the proposed patch-based nonlinear estimation.

Keywords: Dynamic image-guided radiotherapy · Breathing pattern shift · Statistical model-based motion estimation

1 Introduction

In traditional radiation therapy of lung cancer, after obtaining 4D-CT of a patient, the clinical target volume (CTV) and the planned target volume (PTV) are delineated from the average 3D-CT or a selected phase. 4D-CT is used to ensure that PTV covers the tumor during the breathing cycle. The PTV margin can be designed smaller if a gating technology is used during therapy. To better match patient's motion, the radiotherapy

© Springer International Publishing AG 2017
M.J. Cardoso et al. (Eds.): CMMI/RAMBO/SWITCH 2017, LNCS 10555, pp. 55–65, 2017.
DOI: 10.1007/978-3-319-67564-0_6

planning can also be performed in 4D so that radiation can be performed in multiple phases [1–5].

However, it has been found that patient's breathing pattern can change during treatment [6], due to the lack of reproducibility of breathing, or patients tend to calm down or sleep during the treatment. Figure 1 illustrates such variability of breathing using two 4D-CT series of the same subject. We first registered the baseline images (first time-point) of the two image series. After global registration, deformable registration of the two baselines shows large shape differences (mean value of lung field movement range is 12.4 mm (±5.3 mm), and mean value of chest surface movement range is 6.8 mm (±2.6 mm)). Further, the magnitudes of deformation (MOD) of subsequent phases from the respective baseline are plotted. It can be seen that the amounts of breathing are different in the two 4D-CT series. Such breathing trajectory changes in individuals could cause the static planning does not necessarily cover all the breathing cycles well during radiotherapy.

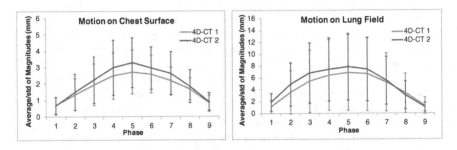

Fig. 1. Magnitudes of deformations (MOD) from baseline (phase 0) to other phases for two 4D-CTs of one subject.

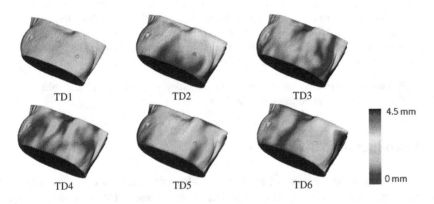

Fig. 2. Different chest motions were observed from the cone-beam CTs for a patient during treatments on different treatment days.

Figure 2 shows examples of MODs of cone-beam CTs captured during six treatments of a subject. TD1 is the surface extracted at treatment day (TD) one. After registering the subsequent TD images to TD1, the magnitudes of deformations (does not count global transformation) are probed on the surface of TD 1 (see TD2-TD6). It can be seen that relatively big differences are close to the armpit, which may be caused by the arm positioning. What is more, patient's breathing statuses are quite different on the chest surfaces, although cone-beam CT images were captured while the patient was freely breathing, and the images reflect different breathing statuses.

These examples indicate that discrepancies between planning-4D-CT images and patient's current breathing pattern could reduce the accuracy for precise treatment. It is in this context that lung motion estimation is particularly useful to adapt the planning-4D-CT onto the patient's current status, and ideally, the real-time respiratory motion can be tracked and compensated by deforming patient's the 4D-CT to his current position. Thus, in this paper, we will study how to estimate the patient's respiratory motion based on one planning-4D-CT of the patient and the real-time measurable chest and upper abdomen signals. The statistics of motion vectors from a population will be used as the prior knowledge for the estimation.

In the literature, surrogate signals, fiducial signals, and surface signals were used for lung motion estimation [7–18]. Specifically, the high-dimensional estimation algorithms indicated that it is possible to estimation lung motion from the chest and abdominal surfaces captured during the radiotherapy procedure. However, these methods attempted to estimate the deformation from one 3D image (e.g., the baseline) to different respiratory phases, and none of them has applied the motion estimation entirely in 4D space.

In this paper, we establish the 4D statistical respiratory model and estimate the lung motion from chest/upper abdomen surface motion sequences. First, we performed statistical analysis on the 4D motion fields, by registering longitudinal motion of each subject onto a patient space. The analysis shows that 4D lung motion is a combination of many complex components, and a limited number of sensor signals might not be sufficient for precise motion estimation. Second, lung respiratory motions are spatially different in the thorax and can be clustered into different partitions. Partitioning of the thorax and estimating the motion within each region under a global smoothness constraint would be more effective to improve the motion estimation accuracy. Finally, both linear and nonlinear estimation algorithms are investigated and compared based on 51 4D-CT datasets.

In experiments, 4D deformation fields of 51 male subjects are used to generate the patch-based Kernel-PCA statistical models. By selecting one subject as the patient to be modeled, all the images are registered onto the patient space. The thorax area is partitioned into 8 regions by applying the K-means clustering algorithm on the normalized longitudinal deformation fields. Then, the statistical model is trained on the patient space, and the lung motion vector of the patient is estimated based on a least-squares optimization method to match the patient's chest and upper abdomen motion. The leave-one-out method was used in the evaluation so that every time 50 subjects were used for the statistical model and 1 subject was used for testing. For each testing subject, we simulated 5 longitudinal deformations from the 4D-CT by sampling from a separate wavelet-based field statistics and tested the estimation from the surfaces extracted. The lung field surface matching accuracy between the estimated images and the original simulated images was calculated. The results suggest that the proposed patch-based

Kernel-PCA estimation improves the performance for lung respiratory motion modeling, and the estimation error is consistently lower than linear and individual phase-based estimation.

2   Method

2.1   Statistical Respiratory Motion Patterns

After intra-subject global registration, 4D-CT of each subject $I^{(s)} = \{I_0^{(s)}, \ldots, I_T^{(s)}\}, s = 1, \ldots, S$ and their longitudinal deformations $\mathbf{f}_{0 \to t}^{(s)}, t = 1, \ldots, T$ are computed using deformable registration [14]. To establish point correspondences across the population, the first time-point or the baseline of each subject $I_0^{(s)}$ is registered to that of the subject p, $I_0^{(p)}$, resulting a global transformation $G_{p \to s}$ and a deformation field $\mathbf{f}_{p \to s}$. Thus, given a voxel $\mathbf{x}$ in p, the motion trajectory for subject s is computed as $\mathbf{m}_{t,\mathbf{x}}^{(s)} = R\big(\mathbf{f}_{p \to s} \circ G_{p \to s}\big)\mathbf{f}_{0 \to t}^{(s)}\big(\mathbf{x} + \mathbf{f}_{p \to s} \circ G_{p \to s}\big), t = 1, \ldots T.$ $\mathbf{x} + \mathbf{f}_{p \to s} \circ G_{p \to s}$ is the corresponding point of $\mathbf{x}$ in the baseline of subject s, and $R\big(\mathbf{f}_{p \to s} \circ G_{p \to s}\big)$ is the rotation matrix of the local Jacobian of the combined global and deformable transformation [9].

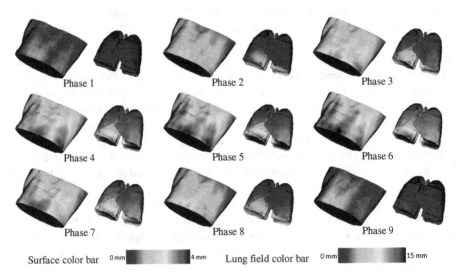

Phase 1   Phase 2   Phase 3

Phase 4   Phase 5   Phase 6

Phase 7   Phase 8   Phase 9

Surface color bar 0 mm ▬▬ 4 mm   Lung field color bar 0 mm ▬▬ 15 mm

Fig. 3. Average motion magnitudes of the population probed on chest and lung field surfaces.

Principal component analysis (PCA) is first computed on the entire 4D motion fields of $S = 50$ subjects, by concatenating the 4D fields of each subject into vectors: $\mathbf{u}^{(s)} = \big[\mathbf{m}_{t,\mathbf{x}}^{(s)T}, \ldots\big]^T$. For all the 50 samples, the magnitudes of the average 4D fields from the baseline chest surface of subject p are shown in Fig. 3. It can be seen that the motion from phase 0 (inhale) reaches the largest at phase 5 (exhale) and comes back at phase 9. The biggest motion appears in the central/lower chest area.

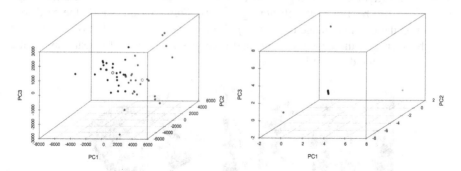

Fig. 4. PCA and Kernel-PCA of 4D lung motion vectors. Left: samples in the three-PC space; and right: samples in the three-Kernel-PC space.

For PCA, the first 10 principal components (PCs) account for 76.7% of the total cumulative variance proportion. Figure 4 left shows the scattered feature points of the first three PCs. Further, the Kernel-PCA of the 50 samples $\mathbf{u}^{(s)}$ is computed, and the projected feature points are shown in Fig. 4 (right). The points are shown in different colors if we cluster them in two (PCA) and four (Kernel-PCA) groups. The figures indicate that respiratory motion patterns are complex and may not be precisely represented linearly by a small number of PCs (Fig. 4 left), and compared to PCA, K-PCA may better represent lung motion pattern variability. To demonstrate different breathing patterns, Fig. 5 shows the motion represented by the two center points (hollow points in Fig. 4, left). In summary, the need of more PCs may explain why surrogate- or fiducial-based estimation has limited ability on precise lung motion estimation because they have limited number of freedom in measuring patient's motion.

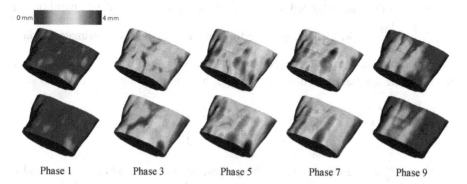

Fig. 5. Two different motion patterns on the template baseline surface based on PCA.

The above statistical lung motion patterns motivate us to improve the statistical representation and estimation performance using nonlinear and patch-based methods:

first, the entire thorax region is partitioned into sub-regions; and then, a Kernel-PCA is applied for the statistical model. For thorax partitioning, the 4D deformation fields are clustered into a number of sub-regions by the K-means algorithm. Further detailed image features can also be used in the clustering [19, 20]. Figure 6 (left) shows the partitions overlaid on the baseline image of subject p. Eight regions were used in our study, and it can be seen that the constraint-free partitioning shows symmetric patterns on the cavity, muscle, and different lung lobes.

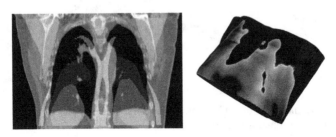

Fig. 6. Lung region partitions and the surface area to be used for motion estimation.

In addition, for the chest surface we threshold the average deformation at phase 5 (see Fig. 3). The highlighted surface area (Fig. 6 right) demonstrates overall motion magnitude larger than 1.8 mm, which will be used in the lung motion estimation, as detailed in next section.

2.2   Patch-Based Linear and Nonlinear Motion Estimation

For a subject s, its entire 4D motion fields can be represented by a vector formed by two parts $[\mathbf{u}^T, \mathbf{v}^T]^T$, with $\mathbf{u}$ as the 4D lung motion fields and $\mathbf{v}$ the corresponding 4D surface motion. $\mathbf{u}$ is partitioned into C parts, so $\mathbf{u} = \cup_{c=1,\ldots,C} \mathbf{u}^c$. Using the method proposed in [21], where a PCA is performed separately for each partition, for the cth partition, we get $\begin{bmatrix} \mathbf{u}^c \\ \mathbf{v} \end{bmatrix} = \begin{bmatrix} \bar{\mathbf{u}}^c \\ \bar{\mathbf{v}} \end{bmatrix} + \mathsf{M}^c\mathbf{b}^c$. The objective for motion estimation is to estimate $\mathbf{u}$ from a given chest motion vector $\mathbf{v}'$, subject to the statistical constraints. This can be achieved by solving the optimal projection vector $\mathbf{b} = \cup_c \mathbf{b}^c$ by minimizing,

$$E(\mathbf{b}) = \sum_{c=1}^{C} \left\{ \left\| \mathbf{v}' - \bar{\mathbf{v}} - \mathsf{M}_v^c\mathbf{b}^c \right\|^2 + \xi \sum_{k=1}^{M} \frac{(b_k^c)^2}{2\lambda_k^c} \right\} + \epsilon \left\| \nabla \cup_c \left(\bar{\mathbf{u}}^c + \mathsf{M}_u^c\mathbf{b}^c \right) \right\|^2. \quad (1)$$

M_u^c and M_v^c are the sub-matrices of M^c, whose rows correspond to vectors $\mathbf{u}$ and $\mathbf{v}$, respectively. The first term ensures the reconstructed surface from the statistical model is similar to the observed one; the second is the statistical prior constraint (M PCs); and the third term is a spatial smoothness constraint for combining different partitions. After solving $\mathbf{b}$ using the finite gradient descent algorithm $\mathbf{u}$ can be estimated.

As discussed in Sect. 2.1, because of the high dimensionality and complexity of lung motion patterns, the relationship between lung motion and surface motion could be better modeled using nonlinear estimation. Herein, we extended the above estimation using Kernel-PCA, which performs PCA after projecting the original data to a high-dimensional space.

For partition c by combining lung motion $\mathbf{u}_c$ with surface motion vector $\mathbf{v}$ into one, i.e., $\mathbf{w}^c = \left[\mathbf{u}^{cT}, \mathbf{v}^T\right]^T$, we can calculate their Kernel-PCA. The radial basis function kernel is used and denoted by $\rho_c(\mathbf{w}^c) = \varkappa(\mathbf{w}^c, \mathbf{w}^c) - 2\sum_{k=1}^{M} b_k^c \sum_{s=1}^{S} \alpha_{k,s}^c \varkappa(\mathbf{w}_s^c, \mathbf{w}^c)$. Denoting K^c as the kernel matrix, by solving the Eigenvalue problem $N\lambda\alpha = K^c\alpha$, we obtain the Eigenvalues λ_k^c and Eigenvectors α_k^c, $k = 1, \ldots, M$ (M is the number of principal components chosen). α_k^c is normalized by $\lambda_k^c\left(\alpha_k^c \cdot \alpha_k^c\right) = 1$. Given a new motion vector of partition c, $\mathbf{w}^c$, the k th element of the projected feature vector $\mathbf{b}^c$ is calculated by,

$$b_k^c = \sum_{s=1,\ldots,S} \alpha_{k,s}^c \varkappa(\mathbf{w}_s^c, \mathbf{w}^c). \tag{2}$$

Because we are interested in a representation of the motion in the original space, not the mapped space, according to [22], given a projection vector $\mathbf{b}^c$, the corresponding motion vector $\mathbf{w}^c$ can be obtained by minimizing $f_c(\mathbf{w}^c) = \sum_{i,j,k} \alpha_{k,i}^c \alpha_{k,j}^c \varkappa(\mathbf{w}_i^c, \mathbf{w}^c)\varkappa(\mathbf{w}_j^c, \mathbf{w}^c)$. On the other hand, the motion vector $\mathbf{w}^c$ needs to be constrained by the shape prior derived from the samples. Different from the multivariate Gaussian prior constraint of PCA, here, the "proximity to data" measure [23] is used. Thus, the shape constraint term is defined by $f_c(\mathbf{w}^c) = \sum_{i,j,k} \alpha_{k,i}^c \alpha_{k,j}^c \varkappa(\mathbf{w}_i^c, \mathbf{w}^c)\varkappa(\mathbf{w}_j^c, \mathbf{w}^c)$. Finally, the surface motion part of $\mathbf{w}^c$, $\mathbf{v}$ needs to be similar with the input surface motion vector $\mathbf{v}'$, and the lung motion vectors $\mathbf{u}^c$ should be spatially smooth across the partition boundaries. Combining these requirements, we come up with the following objective function:

$$E(\mathbf{w}) = \sum_{c=1,\ldots,C} \left\{ \rho_c(\mathbf{w}^c) + \varepsilon f_c(\mathbf{w}^c) + \eta\left\|\mathbf{v} - \mathbf{v}'\right\|^2 + \epsilon\left\|\nabla_c\mathbf{u}\right\|^2 \right\}. \tag{3}$$

In short, the first term is the Kernel-PCA reconstruction, the second is the prior constraint, the third is the similarity between the actual surface signal and the one generated from the statistical model, and the last term is smoothness across different partitions. The finite gradient method can be used to optimize Eq. (3). We iteratively calculate $\mathbf{b}$ using Eq. (2) after each optimization of Eq. (3) until the differences of $\mathbf{w}$ in two consequent iterations are smaller than a prescribed threshold. Notice that the initial values of $\mathbf{u}_c$ are unknown, and we set them to the mean of the S samples.

3   Results

The linear and nonlinear estimation algorithms were implemented using R and performed on a server with 24 cores and 32 GB memory running Ubuntu 16.04 × 64. Slicer software was used for visualization. 51 4D-CT of male lung cancer patients undergoing radiotherapy were used. The exception is Fig. 2, where a female data was illustrated due to availability. In the future, we will evaluate/eliminate the effects of the breast area and study whether it is feasible to combine both genders. Only subjects with small lesions <5 cm are selected. Each data has 10 respiratory phases: the first (baseline) is inhale; the 5th is exhale; the 9th is inhale, representing a breathing cycle. The in-plane resolution is 1.17 mm and the slice thickness is 3 mm for all the images.

To evaluate the performance, we used the leave-one-out strategy. In each test, the real 4D-CT, as well as simulated longitudinal deformations for the testing subject, were used as ground truth: 5 image series were randomly sampled from the wavelet-based deformation statistics trained without the testing subject. Different bands of the wavelet coefficients were independently sampled so the simulation is a mimic of piece-wise linear simulation. Please refer to [24] for more details. The reason for simulating image series is to test the algorithm on more breathing variability with known "ground truth". Chest surfaces for each image series were extracted by deforming the chest surface of the template baseline onto them, and the serial surfaces act as the input surface signals $\mathbf{v}'$. Because no global transformation was simulated, it was not considered in the experiments. Altogether, we generated 6×51 testing data (1 real + 5 simulated for each leave-one-out study) and estimated the corresponding 4D-CT images using linear and nonlinear estimation, respectively.

We compared the linear, nonlinear, and the single-phase-based 3D estimation [9] – images of individual phases were estimated directly from the baseline. Parameters ε, η, and ϵ were selected so that the second term contribute half, and the third and fourth terms contribute ¼ of the initial values of the first term. Surface distances between the lung field surfaces extracted from the testing images and those extracted from the estimated image sequences were calculated as the measure of the results [25].

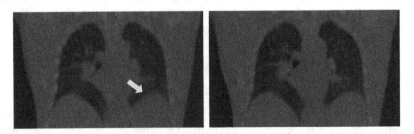

Fig. 7. Overlay of estimated image on original image (left: linear; right: nonlinear estimation). (Color figure online)

Figure 7 shows an example of the reconstructed image (red) overlaid on the testing image (gray scale) for phase 5. In Fig. 8, the average and std of the differences for each phase over all the 306 tests are plotted. We can see that nonlinear estimation performed better compared to linear methodology. Notably, unlike the individual phase-based estimation which estimates the deformation from baseline to different phases and yields larger error when the breathing motion is large, by modeling the statistics and estimation in 4D, the estimation error turns to be stable across different phases. We plan to perform a further evaluation on multiple real 4D-CT images for patients who need repeated 4D-CT scans. Currently, estimation can be accomplished within 10 min, but parallel computing and pre-computation of multiple image series may boost onsite evaluation in operation.

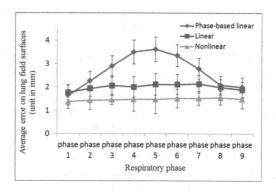

Fig. 8. Average estimation errors on lung field surfaces.

4   Conclusion

The lack of reproducibility of respiratory motion limits breathing motion pattern shifts for patients undergoing lung cancer treatment. In this paper, we propose to dynamically align planning-4D-CT onto patient space by adapting to the real-time collectible chest surface motion. Partition-based 4D breathing statistics of a population are applied as priors in motion estimation. The comparative results with 51 4D-CTs showed that nonlinear estimation outperforms the linear method and also yields consistently smaller errors for different phases.

References

1. Tachibana, H., Sawant, A.: Four-dimensional planning for motion synchronized dose delivery in lung stereotactic body radiation therapy. Radiother. Oncol. **119**, 467–472 (2016)
2. Wilms, M., Werner, R., Blendowski, M., Ortmuller, J., Handels, H.: Simulation of range imaging-based estimation of respiratory lung motion. Influence of noise, signal dimensionality and sampling patterns. Methods Inf. Med. **53**, 257–263 (2014)
3. Rottmann, J., Keall, P., Berbeco, R.: Real-time soft tissue motion estimation for lung tumors during radiotherapy delivery. Med. Phys. **40**, 091713 (2013)
4. Dong, B., Graves, Y.J., Jia, X., Jiang, S.B.: Optimal surface marker locations for tumor motion estimation in lung cancer radiotherapy. Phys. Med. Biol. **57**, 8201–8215 (2012)
5. Liu, X., Saboo, R.R., Pizer, S.M., Mageras, G.S.: A shape-navigated image deformation model for 4d lung respiratory motion estimation. In: Proceedings of IEEE International Symposium on Biomedical Imaging 2009, pp. 875–878 (2009)
6. Takao, S., Miyamoto, N., Matsuura, T., Onimaru, R., Katoh, N., Inoue, T., Sutherland, K.L., Suzuki, R., Shirato, H., Shimizu, S.: Intrafractional baseline shift or drift of lung tumor motion during gated radiation therapy with a real-time tumor-tracking system. Int. J. Radiat. Oncol. Biol. Phys. **94**, 172–180 (2016)

7. Ehrhardt, J., Werner, R., Schmidt-Richberg, A., Handels, H.: Statistical modeling of 4D respiratory lung motion using diffeomorphic image registration. IEEE Trans. Med. Imaging **30**, 251–265 (2011)

8. Han, D., Bayouth, J., Song, Q., Bhatia, S., Sonka, M., Wu, X.: Feature guided motion artifact reduction with structure-awareness in 4D CT images. In: IEEE Conference on Computer Vision and Pattern Recognition (CVPR), pp. 1057–1064. IEEE (2011)

9. He, T., Xue, Z., Yu, N., Nitsch, P.L., Teh, B.S., Wong, S.T.: Estimating dynamic lung images from high-dimension chest surface motion using 4D statistical model. Med. Image Comput. Comput. Assist. Interv. **17**, 138–145 (2014)

10. Klinder, T., Lorenz, C., Ostermann, J.: Prediction framework for statistical respiratory motion modeling. Med. Image Comput. Comput. Assist. Interv. **13**, 327–334 (2010)

11. Lu, W., Song, J.H., Christensen, G.E., Parikh, P.J., Zhao, T., Hubenschmidt, J.P., Bradley, J.D., Low, D.A.: Evaluating lung motion variations in repeated 4D CT studies using inverse consistent image registration. Int. J. Radiat. Oncol. Biol. Phys. **66**, S606–S607 (2006)

12. Santelli, C., Nezafat, R., Goddu, B., Manning, W.J., Smink, J., Kozerke, S., Peters, D.C.: Respiratory bellows revisited for motion compensation: preliminary experience for cardiovascular MR. Magn. Reson. Med. **65**, 1098–1103 (2011)

13. Vandemeulebroucke, J., Rit, S., Kybic, J., Clarysse, P., Sarrut, D.: Spatiotemporal motion estimation for respiratory-correlated imaging of the lungs. Med. Phys. **38**, 166–178 (2011)

14. Wu, G., Wang, Q., Lian, J., Shen, D.: Estimating the 4D respiratory lung motion by spatiotemporal registration and building super-resolution image. Med. Image Comput. Comput. Assist. Interv. **14**, 532–539 (2011)

15. Zeng, R., Fessler, J.A., Balter, J.M., Balter, P.A.: Iterative sorting for 4DCT images based on internal anatomy motion. In: 4th IEEE International Symposium on Biomedical Imaging, pp. 744–747. IEEE (2007)

16. Yang, D., Lu, W., Low, D.A., Deasy, J.O., Hope, A.J., El Naqa, I.: 4D-CT motion estimation using deformable image registration and 5D respiratory motion modeling. Med. Phys. **35**, 4577–4590 (2008)

17. Lu, B., Chen, Y., Park, J.C., Fan, Q., Kahler, D., Liu, C.: A method of surface marker location optimization for tumor motion estimation in lung stereotactic body radiation therapy. Med. Phys. **42**, 244–253 (2015)

18. Wilms, M., Werner, R., Yamamoto, T., Handels, H., Ehrhardt, J.: Subpopulation-based correspondence modelling for improved respiratory motion estimation in the presence of inter-fraction motion variations. Phys. Med. Biol. **62**, 5823–5839 (2017)

19. Heinrich, M.P., Jenkinson, M., Papież, B.W., Glesson, F.V., Brady, S.M., Schnabel, J.A.: Edge- and detail-preserving sparse image representations for deformable registration of chest MRI and CT volumes. In: Gee, J.C., Joshi, S., Pohl, K.M., Wells, W.M., Zöllei, L. (eds.) IPMI 2013. LNCS, vol. 7917, pp. 463–474. Springer, Heidelberg (2013). doi:10.1007/978-3-642-38868-2_39

20. Papież, B.W., Franklin, J., Heinrich, M.P., Gleeson, F.V., Schnabel, J.A.: Liver motion estimation via locally adaptive over-segmentation regularization. In: Navab, N., Hornegger, J., Wells, W.M., Frangi, A.F. (eds.) MICCAI 2015. LNCS, vol. 9351, pp. 427–434. Springer, Cham (2015). doi:10.1007/978-3-319-24574-4_51

21. Xue, Z., Pino, R., Teh, B.: Estimating lung respiratory motion using combined global and local statistical models. In: Wu, G., Coupé, P., Zhan, Y., Munsell, B.C., Rueckert, D. (eds.) Patch-MI 2016. LNCS, vol. 9993, pp. 133–140. Springer, Cham (2016). doi:10.1007/978-3-319-47118-1_17

22. Schölkopf, B., Mika, S., Smola, A., Rätsch, G., Müller, K.-R.: Kernel PCA pattern reconstruction via approximate pre-images. In: Niklasson, L., Bodén, M., Ziemke, T. (eds.) ICANN 98, pp. 147–152. Springer, London (1998)

23. Twining, C.J., Taylor, C.J.: Kernel principal component analysis and the construction of non-linear active shape models. In: BMVC, pp. 23–32. (2001)
24. Davatzikos, C., Tao, X., Shen, D.: Hierarchical active shape models, using the wavelet transform. IEEE Trans. Med. Imaging **22**, 414–423 (2003)
25. Gerig, G., Jomier, M., Chakos, M.: Valmet: a new validation tool for assessing and improving 3D object segmentation. In: Niessen, W.J., Viergever, M.A. (eds.) MICCAI 2001. LNCS, vol. 2208, pp. 516–523. Springer, Heidelberg (2001). doi:10.1007/3-540-45468-3_62

Mass Transportation for Deformable Image Registration with Application to Lung CT

Bartłomiej W. Papież[1]([✉]), Sir Michael Brady[2], and Julia A. Schnabel[1,3]

[1] Department of Engineering Science, Institute of Biomedical Engineering,
University of Oxford, Oxford, UK
bartlomiej.papiez@eng.ox.ac.uk
[2] Department of Oncology, University of Oxford, Oxford, UK
[3] Department of Biomedical Engineering, Division of Imaging Sciences and
Biomedical Engineering, King's College London, London, UK

Abstract. Computed Tomography (CT) of the lungs play a key role in clinical investigation of thoracic malignancies, as well as having the potential to increase our knowledge about pulmonary diseases including cancer. It enables longitudinal trials to monitor lung disease progression, and to inform assessment of lung damage resulting from radiation therapy. We present a novel deformable image registration method that accommodates changes in the density of lung tissue depending on the amount of air present in the lungs inspiration/expiration state. We investigate the Monge-Kantorovich theory of optimal mass transportation to model the appearance of lung tissue and apply it in a method for registration. To validate the model, we apply our method to an inhale and exhale lung CT data set, and compare it against registration using the sum of squared differences (SSD) as a representative of the most popular similarity measures used in deformable image registration. The results show that the developed registration method has the potential to handle intensity distortions caused by air and tissue compression, and in addition it can provide accurate annotations of the lungs.

1 Introduction

Deformable image registration (DIR) of Computed Tomography (CT) images of the lungs is used in a range of clinical applications including diagnosis and radiation therapy. For instance, longitudinal DIR of CT images helps to monitor and visualize disease progression including lung nodule changes, radiotherapy planning, and/or regional lung ventilation. Consequently, DIR methods have become increasingly important in informing clinicians and in supporting medical physicists in quantitative analyses of data sets, by presenting them in a common coordinate frame. The estimation of *plausible* correspondences between data sets is a crucial step in analyzing longitudinal data [6]. It is particularly challenging in clinical trials where data may be acquired several weeks apart. As usual, the choice of the similarity measure in the DIR method plays a key role, since it describes the (dis)similarity between the images to be registered.

© Springer International Publishing AG 2017
M.J. Cardoso et al. (Eds.): CMMI/RAMBO/SWITCH 2017, LNCS 10555, pp. 66–74, 2017.
DOI: 10.1007/978-3-319-67564-0_7

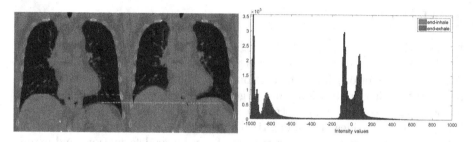

Fig. 1. Coronal view for (left) inhale and exhale lung CTs, and (right) their corresponding intensity distributions showing significant changes in tissue density due to large volume change over the breathing cycle. The difference in lung volume is highlighted by magenta and green lines. (Color figure online)

Typical choices, such as the sum of the squared differences (SSD), assume that anatomical locations deemed to be in correspondence are represented by the same intensity value. However, this assumption is invalid when the task is to register lung CT volumes that are acquired at different breathing phases, since in such cases the lung tissue density is related to the amount of air present in the lungs (see Fig. 1). This is despite the fact that CT voxels are given as Hounsfield Units (HU), which, unlike image intensities in ultrasound and magnetic resonance imaging (MRI), are physical parameters that measure the X-ray attenuation of the tissue. Local changes intensity may also indicate the effectiveness of radiation therapy [5]. Intensity changes resulting from tissue compression have previously been considered in the literature using mass preserving DIR [7,20]. Both [7,20] modeled lung tissue density using the determinant of the Jacobian of the transformation function. Since the density of lungs is inversely proportional to the local volume, the local volume change can be estimated from the change in density.

Contributions. We explore optimal mass transportation to lung CT volumes as a method that is intrinsically invariant to lung expiration/inspiration, and thus lung tissue density. In particular, we developed a joint segmentation and registration approach using optimal mass transportation theory to enable assessment of lung CT intensity changes. The main contributions of this manuscript are as follows: we use the Wasserstein distance to measure the similarity between local HU distributions (represented as histograms) for joint segmentation and registration. We do this because the Wassserstein distance is a closed-form solution to the optimal mass transport equations when the distributions are one-dimensional. Local distributions (histogram) representations, and the Wasserstein distance, are combined within a level-set framework to deal effectively with: changes in local tissue properties; significant levels of noise; and image acquisition artifacts.

2   Methods

We first describe our general joint registration and segmentation framework, which extends the idea of level set registration [17], and level set segmentation [3]. A number of joint segmentation and registration approaches have been reported for other applications, and in general they show improved performance for both segmentation and registration e.g. for human lungs [15,16]. Yezzi et al. [19] introduced the idea of coupling rigid registration and segmentation within an active contours framework. Incorporation of non-linear deformations and extension to a 3D segmentation model, which was the main limiting factor of this approach was presented in [8]. Recently this variational formulation has been extended to 4D image time series of dynamic contrast-enhanced magnetic resonance imaging (DCE-MRI), where respiratory-induced motion was compensated for in parallel with multi-compartment kidney segmentation [10].

Level Set Deformation Fields (LSDF). For segmentation, we consider general Chan-Vese level set formulation [3]. Our choice of formulation comes from the fact that level-sets have been used as a well-known example to illustrate the mass transportation idea, however it would be relatively straightforward to extend to any other segmentation and registration framework. First, we define a contour Γ in the image domain Ω to be the boundary distinguishing between the areas Ω_1 (e.g. inside the contour Γ) and $\Omega_2 = \Omega \setminus \Omega_1$ (e.g. outside the contour Γ). The key idea as regards to segmentation is to evolve the contour Γ from its given initial position in the direction of minimizing the cost function ε_{seg}:

$$\frac{\partial \Gamma}{\partial t} = -\frac{\partial \varepsilon_{seg}(\Gamma)}{\partial \Gamma} \tag{1}$$

Following [3,4], the contour Γ can be represented as the zero level set of a function Φ: $\Gamma = \{x \in \Omega \mid \Phi(x) = 0\}$, and the evolution equation (Eq. (1)) is then defined on the space of the level set function:

$$\frac{\partial \Phi}{\partial t} = -\frac{\partial \varepsilon_{seg}(\Phi)}{\partial \Phi} = -F\frac{\nabla \Phi}{|\nabla \Phi|} \tag{2}$$

where F is a speed function, and $\frac{\nabla \Phi}{|\nabla \Phi|}$ defines the normal direction of the level set contour evolution. Chan and Vese [3] proposed the following cost function for a binary (two phase) segmentation ε_{seg}:

$$\arg\min_{\Omega_1, \Omega_2} \left(\varepsilon_{seg}(\Omega_1, \Omega_2) = \int_{\Omega_1} \rho(x, \mu_1)dx + \int_{\Omega_2} \rho(x, \mu_2)dx + \kappa|\Gamma| \right) \tag{3}$$

where μ_1 and μ_2 are the mean values of the areas Ω_1 and Ω_2, respectively, and the final term of Eq. (3) represents the constraint that minimizes the length of the contour.

As well as segmentation, we also consider pair-wise image registration between two 3D CT volumes, namely the reference image I_R and source image I_S.

Deformable image registration (DIR) process aims to estimate a plausible transformation φ represented by dense deformation field $\boldsymbol{u}$: $\varphi(\boldsymbol{x}) = \boldsymbol{x} + \boldsymbol{u}(\boldsymbol{x})$, where $\boldsymbol{x}$ is spatial coordinate. A generic non-linear registration framework can be formulated as the minimization of a cost functional ε_{reg} as follows:

$$\arg \min_{\boldsymbol{u}} \left(\varepsilon_{reg}\left(\boldsymbol{u}\right) = D(I_R, I_S(\boldsymbol{u})) + \gamma R(\boldsymbol{u}) \right) \tag{4}$$

where ε combines a (dis)similarity between input images D and R is some suitable regularization term. The original idea of Vemuri's registration framework [17] to address the registration problem (given by Eq. (4)) is to solve a partial differential equation of level set intensity evolution with explicit tracking of the deformation field $\boldsymbol{u}$ as follows:

$$\frac{d\boldsymbol{u}(\boldsymbol{x}, t)}{dt} = F(\boldsymbol{x}, t) \frac{\nabla I_S(\boldsymbol{x}, t)}{\|\nabla I_S(\boldsymbol{x}, t)\|} \tag{5}$$

where $F(\boldsymbol{x}, t)$ is the speed function, which was defined in [17] as an intensity difference $(I_S(\boldsymbol{x}, t) - I_R(\boldsymbol{x}))$, and $\nabla I_S(\boldsymbol{x}, t)$ is the direction of the intensity based level set evolution at spatial position $\boldsymbol{x}$ and at time t. The warped image at time t, which we denote by $I_S(\boldsymbol{u}) = I_S\left(\boldsymbol{x} + \boldsymbol{u}(\boldsymbol{x}, t)\right)$, is given by warping the source image I_S using the deformation field $\boldsymbol{u}$. By coupling the level set evolution equation for segmentation (given by Eq. (3)) with the deformation field $\boldsymbol{u}$: $\rho(\boldsymbol{x} + \boldsymbol{u}(\boldsymbol{x}), \mu)$, one obtains the level set deformation field framework for joint registration and segmentation [8]:

$$\arg \min_{\boldsymbol{u}} \left(\alpha \varepsilon_{reg}\left(\boldsymbol{u}\right) + \beta \varepsilon_{seg}\left(\boldsymbol{u}\right) \right) \tag{6}$$

where α and β are user-defined parameters balancing between registration and segmentation. Equation (6) indicates that registration is driven both by the registration term ε_{reg} and the segmentation term ε_{seg}, so the estimated displacement field $\boldsymbol{u}$ maximizes the matching between objects of interest in the reference image and the warped source image.

Locally Optimal Mass Transportation. The mass transport problem investigates ways to find the optimal redistribution of mass [9]. A solution to the optimal transportation problem is given by the Monge-Kantorovich theorem and such defines it as a minimal cost transforming one probability density function (*pdf*) into another. In the case of CT volumes, we can approximate a *pdf* for the intensities by calculating a local intensity histogram $h_p(\boldsymbol{x})$ at each spatial position $\boldsymbol{x} \in \Omega_I$ within a local neighborhood p. In the special case of one-dimensional histograms with equally weighted bins, the Wasserstein distance (viz. the Earth Mover Distance [14]) is simplified to a closed-form solution of optimal mass transport, which is defined as follows:

$$\rho_W(h_1, h_2) = \sum_{b=1}^{B} \left(|cdf_1(b) - cdf_2(b)| \right) \tag{7}$$

where cdf_1 and cdf_2 are the cumulative distribution functions of the local histograms h_1 and h_2 respectively, and B is the number of bins used for the histogram calculation. In the context of lung segmentation and registration, the use of a non-parametric model based on local histograms has yet another advantage because it makes no assumptions either about the image intensity distribution or the type of noise. In CT, intensity values correspond to Hounsfield Units (HU), which represent the radiological density of the tissue, and while this is not the same as biomechanical density, for the lung they are closely correlated. This is because for a CT of the lungs it may be assumed that the lung comprises two compartments: tissue (parenchyma and blood) and air [20]. Based on these observations, our DIR method is explicitly driven by the Wasserstein distance between local histograms. The energy function can be formulated within the Chan-Vese level set method as a minimization problem of finding an optimal region e.g. Ω_i represented by local histogram h_1 as follows:

$$\arg \min_{\Omega_1, \Omega_2} \left(\varepsilon_{seg} \left(\Omega_1, \Omega_2 \right) = \int_{\Omega_1} \rho_W(h_1, h(\boldsymbol{x})) d\boldsymbol{x} + \int_{\Omega_2} \rho_W(h_2, h(\boldsymbol{x})) d\boldsymbol{x} \right) \quad (8)$$

where $h(\boldsymbol{x})$ is a local histogram that depends only on the spatial location $\boldsymbol{x}$, and can therefore be computed efficiently before registration (see implementation details in Sect. 3). Similarly, the approximation of the histograms for the regions of interest h_i is not a function of the displacement field $\boldsymbol{u}$, so it can remain fixed during optimization.

It may be argued that a multimodal similarity measure such as joint entropy or mutual information are both estimated based on a *pdf* and so may capture changes to the intensity values in lung CT. However, we require the measurement to represent tissue density distributions, as part of a mass transportation algorithm, to model density changes associated with lung inflation, and this is less obviously the case for conventional *pdf*-based similarity measures.

Diffeomorphic LSDF. In order to preserve the smoothness of the estimated displacement field $\boldsymbol{u}$, parameterization of the contour evolution is done via iterative estimation of the final displacement field $\hat{\boldsymbol{u}}$ defined as follows:

$$\hat{\boldsymbol{u}} = \boldsymbol{u}_1 + \ldots + \boldsymbol{u}_n + \ldots + \boldsymbol{u}_N \quad (9)$$

where n is an iteration index, and N is the maximum number of iterations. However, addition of partial estimates of the displacement field $\boldsymbol{u}_n$ may potentially lead to undesired effects such as folding or tearing of the displacement field [18]. In many biomedical applications, including lung assessment presented in this paper, such a lack of one-to-one correspondence between the registered volumes is considered to be implausible. In order to preserve the regional topology of organs, we parameterize the evolution of the contour encoded as the displacement field $\boldsymbol{u}$ in terms of exponential mapping of a stationary velocity field $\boldsymbol{u} = \exp(\boldsymbol{v})$ using approximation of a Lie group structure on diffeomorphism (see details in [1]). Such a representation of the displacement field brings significant benefits.

First, it constrains the estimated deformation field $\hat{\boldsymbol{u}}$ to be diffeomorphic (so preserves the one-to-one mapping between the regions of interest). Second, the exponential mapping can easily be calculated using a recursive scale-and-square algorithm [1], resulting in an overall efficient implementation of a diffeomorphic level set deformation field framework. In summary, the diffeomorphic evolution of the contour is calculated as follows:

$$\frac{d\boldsymbol{v}(\boldsymbol{x}, t)}{dt} = F(\boldsymbol{x}, t) \frac{\nabla I_S(\boldsymbol{x}, t)}{\|\nabla I_S(\boldsymbol{x}, t)\|} \tag{10}$$

and the final diffeomorphic displacement field is estimated by:

$$\hat{\boldsymbol{u}} = \exp(\boldsymbol{v}_1) \circ \ldots \circ \exp(\boldsymbol{v}_n) \circ \ldots \circ \exp(\boldsymbol{v}_N) \tag{11}$$

where $\circ$ denotes an composition operator. Calculation of updates on the Lie algebra mapped through the exponential mapping has been previously considered for non-linear dense registration e.g. in [18]. In contrast, here we propose to use it as a constraint for contour evolution in a joint registration and segmentation framework. Thus, due to the assumption of the diffeomorphic evolution of the contour, we exclude from our approach the explicit contour constraint $\kappa|\Gamma|$ from the cost function (given by Eq. (3)).

3 Experiments and Results

Numerical Implementation. While the specifics of implementation are not the primary focus of this article, the following details should enable any interested reader to reproduce our work. First, the new similarity measure (the Wasserstein distance) and diffeomorphic contour propagation have been incorporated into the level-set approach (see details in [17]). Following [17], the images were smoothed with a Gaussian kernel because of image noise. For regularization, we chose isotropic Gaussian smoothing of the displacement field [18]. The composition of the exponential mapping (Eq. (11)) for contour propagation is approximated using the Baker-Campbell-Hausdorff formula (see details in [1]). The Euler-Lagrange equations for the Wasserstein based contour evolution are as presented in [12]. As an efficient method of calculating local histograms with different patch sizes we used a concept of so-called *integral* images (or histograms) proposed in [13]. A size of patch to calculate local histogram from integral images is $7 \times 7 \times 7$. The contour is initialized prior to registration based on labels obtained from manual delineation of the baseline volumes.

Data Description. We have evaluated our method using a publicly available 4D CT data set [2]. The *Dir-Lab* data set consists of 10 consecutive respiratory cycle phase volumes with spatial resolution varying between $0.97 \times 0.97 \times 2.5$ and $1.16 \times 1.16 \times 2.5$ mm^3. To quantify the registration accuracy, we calculated the Target Registration Error (TRE) for the well-distributed set of landmarks, which are provided with this data set (300 landmarks per case for inhale and exhale volumes). In all cases, the end-inhale image was selected as the baseline image and the end-exhale image as the moving image.

Experimental Setup. We compare our method against the state-of-the-art level-set registration methods: (**vem**) Vemuri's level set registration [17], (**c-v**) Chan-Vese segmentation driven registration (following implementation details given in [8]), and (**our**) registration with local mass transportation model.

Results. The initial TRE is 8.46 ± 5.5 mm and the transformations estimated by the proposed method (**our**) reduce the TRE to 2.64 ± 2.2 mm, achieving the best result in our comparison. Vemuri's level set registration [17] reduces the TRE to 2.72 ± 2.2 mm, and finally (**c-v**) Chan-Vese [8] segmentation driven registration achieves the TRE to 3.40 ± 1.1 mm. The TRE achieved by our proposed method is slightly lower than the TRE for Vemuri's method. This can be however explained by the level of inspiration/expiration, which is relatively low in this data set.

Visualization of the results for the presented method is shown in Fig. 2. While both methods produce similar TRE, Vemuri's method does not distribute density across the lung region, whereas our method gives results that match well density distributions within the lung region. Our results are consistent with the results from [7], where only minor improvement in terms of the TRE was found.

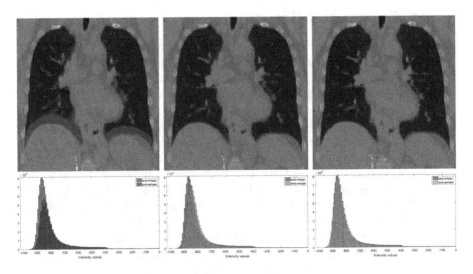

Fig. 2. Coronal view of differences between inhale and exhale CTs and their corresponding intensity distributions calculated within the lung region only: (left) before registration, after registration using: (middle) Vemuri's level set registration (**vem**) based on the SSD, and (right) (**our**) method with locally optimal mass transportation model. Our method successfully models density changes associated with lung inflation.

4 Discussion and Conclusions

In this paper, we have investigated the use of optimal transportation theory for deformable image registration of lung CT. We incorporated the Wasserstein distance, which is a solution to optimal transportation problem, as a similarity measure to our DIR using level-set framework. We evaluated our method on pairs of CT images acquired over breathing cycle, in which there are intensity changes due lung tissue compression. Our initial results suggest that our model can handle such tissue density changes in a plausible way. Future work is focused on evaluation of our method for longitudinal clinical studies of lung disease progression including publicly available thoracic CT data (EMPIRE10) [11] and assessment of radiation induced lung injuries.

Acknowledgments. We would like to acknowledge funding from the CRUK/ EPSRC Cancer Imaging Centre in Oxford.

References

1. Arsigny, V., Commowick, O., Pennec, X., Ayache, N.: A log-euclidean framework for statistics on diffeomorphisms. In: Larsen, R., Nielsen, M., Sporring, J. (eds.) MICCAI 2006. LNCS, vol. 4190, pp. 924–931. Springer, Heidelberg (2006). doi:10.1007/11866565_113
2. Castillo, R., Castillo, E., Guerra, R., Johnson, V., McPhail, T., Garg, A., Guerrero, T.: A framework for evaluation of deformable image registration spatial accuracy using large landmark point sets. Phys. Med. Biol. **54**, 1849–1870 (2009)
3. Chan, T.F., Vese, L.A.: Active contours without edges. IEEE Trans. Image Process. **10**(2), 266–277 (2001)
4. Cremers, D., Rousson, M., Deriche, R.: A review of statistical approaches to level set segmentation: integrating color, texture, motion and shape. Int. J. Comput. Vision **72**(2), 195–215 (2007)
5. Dawson, L.A., Jaffray, D.A.: Advances in image-guided radiation therapy. J. Clin. Oncol. **25**(8), 938–946 (2007)
6. Durrleman, S., Pennec, X., Trouvé, A., Braga, J., Gerig, G., Ayache, N.: Toward a comprehensive framework for the spatiotemporal statistical analysis of longitudinal shape data. Int. J. Comput. Vision **103**(1), 22–59 (2013)
7. Gorbunova, V., Sporring, J., Lo, P., Loeve, M., Tiddens, H.A., Nielsen, M., Dirksen, A., de Bruijne, M.: Mass preserving image registration for lung CT. Med. Image Anal. **16**(4), 786–795 (2012)
8. Gorthi, S., Duay, V., Bresson, X., Cuadra, M., Castro, F.S., Pollo, C., Allal, A., Thiran, J.-P.: Active deformation fields: dense deformation field estimation for atlas-based segmentation using the active contour framework. Med. Image Anal. **15**(6), 787–800 (2011)
9. Haker, S., Zhu, L., Tannenbaum, A., Angenent, S.: Optimal mass transport for registration and warping. Int. J. Comput. Vision **60**(3), 225–240 (2004)
10. Hodneland, E., Hanson, E., Lundervold, A., Modersitzki, J., Eikefjord, E., Munthe-Kaas, A.: Segmentation-driven image registration-application to 4D DCE-MRI recordings of the moving kidneys. IEEE Trans. Image Process (2014)

11. Murphy, K., Van Ginneken, B., Reinhardt, J.M., Kabus, S., Ding, K., Deng, X., Cao, K., Du, K., Christensen, G.E., Garcia, V., et al.: Evaluation of registration methods on thoracic CT: the EMPIRE10 challenge. IEEE Trans. Med. Imaging **30**(11), 1901–1920 (2011)
12. Ni, K., Bresson, X., Chan, T.F., Esedoglu, S.: Local histogram based segmentation using the Wasserstein distance. Int. J. Comput. Vision **84**, 97–111 (2009)
13. Porikli, F.M.: Integral histogram: a fast way to extract histograms in cartesian spaces. In: IEEE Computer Society Conference on Computer Vision and Pattern Recognition, vol. 1, pp. 829–836. IEEE (2005)
14. Rubner, Y., Tomasi, C., Leonidas, J.G.: The earth movers distance as a metric for image retrieval. Int. J. Comput. Vision **40**, 99–121 (2000)
15. Świerczyński, P., Papież, B.W., Schnabel, J.A., Macdonald, C.: A level-set approach to joint image segmentation and registration with application to CT lung imaging. Comput. Med. Imaging Graph. (2017, in press)
16. Vandemeulebroucke, J., Bernard, O., Rit, S., Kybic, J., Clarysse, P., Sarrut, D.: Automated segmentation of a motion mask to preserve sliding motion in deformable registration of thoracic CT. Med. Phys. **39**, 1006 (2012)
17. Vemuri, B.C., Ye, J., Chen, Y., Leonard, C.M.: Image registration via level-set motion: applications to atlas-based segmentation. Med. Image Anal. **7**, 1–20 (2003)
18. Vercauteren, T., Pennec, X., Perchant, A., Ayache, N.: Diffeomorphic demons: efficient non-parametric image registration. Neuroimage **45**, S61–S72 (2009)
19. Yezzi, A., Zöllei, L., Kapur, T.: A variational framework for integrating segmentation and registration through active contours. Med. Image Anal. **7**, 171–18 (2003)
20. Yin, Y., Hoffman, E.A., Lin, C.-L.: Mass preserving nonrigid registration of CT lung images using cubic B-spline. Med. Phys. **36**(9), 4213–4222 (2009)

Motion-Robust Spatially Constrained Parameter Estimation in Renal Diffusion-Weighted MRI by 3D Motion Tracking and Correction of Sequential Slices

Sila Kurugol[(✉)], Bahram Marami, Onur Afacan, Simon K. Warfield, and Ali Gholipour

Department of Radiology, Boston Children's Hospital, Harvard Medical School, Boston, USA
sila.kurugol@childrens.harvard.edu

Abstract. In this work, we introduce a novel motion-robust spatially constrained parameter estimation (MOSCOPE) technique for kidney diffusion-weighted MRI. The proposed motion compensation technique does not require a navigator, trigger, or breath-hold but only uses the intrinsic features of the acquired data to track and compensate for motion to reconstruct precise models of the renal diffusion signal. We have developed a technique for physiological motion tracking based on robust state estimation and sequential registration of diffusion sensitized slices acquired within 200 ms. This allows a sampling rate of 5 Hz for state estimation in motion tracking that is sufficiently faster than both respiratory and cardiac motion rates in children and adults, which range between 0.8 to 0.2 Hz, and 2.5 to 1 Hz, respectively. We then apply the estimated motion parameters to data from each slice and use motion-compensated data for (1) robust intra-voxel incoherent motion (IVIM) model estimation in the kidney using a spatially constrained model fitting approach, and (2) robust weighted least squares estimation of the diffusion tensor model. Experimental results, including precision of IVIM model parameters using bootstrap-sampling and *in-vivo* whole kidney tractography, showed significant improvement in precision and accuracy of these models using the proposed method compared to models based on the original data and volumetric registration.

1 Introduction

Quantitative diffusion-weighted MRI (DW-MRI) of kidneys has shown to be useful in evaluating renal microstructure and function in clinical applications such as renal fibrosis and allograft dysfunction [4]. The kidney is a highly perfused organ with complex anatomy including multiple compartments with isotropic (cortex) and anisotropic (medulla) diffusion properties. Accurate model fitting and estimation of IVIM [16] parameters of slow diffusion (due to Brownian motion) and fast diffusion (due to microcapillary perfusion and flow), as well as parameters

© Springer International Publishing AG 2017
M.J. Cardoso et al. (Eds.): CMMI/RAMBO/SWITCH 2017, LNCS 10555, pp. 75–85, 2017.
DOI: 10.1007/978-3-319-67564-0_8

of diffusion anisotropy is limited by several factors. The physiological motion including respiratory and cardiac motion, and low signal-to-noise-ratio (SNR) reduces the reliability of estimated model parameters. Especially, the estimation of the micro-capillary perfusion contribution has demonstrated a large variability [4], which is considered to be largely due to uncompensated (residual) motion.

Navigator triggering, breath-holding, 3D rigid or 2D slice-based registration techniques have been used for motion compensation in renal DW-MRI [14,23]. Recent studies demonstrate the impact of motion compensation; however, current motion compensation techniques either require a complex setup (breath-holding, external devices), increase scan time (triggering, respiratory gating), or cannot fully correct for the effect of motion (e.g., gating, and 3D volumetric registration, or 2D slice-based registration). Respiratory gating prolongs scan time and does not use the entire data. Breath-holding prolongs scan times and cannot be used in patients who cannot hold their breath, for example young children. In this work, we propose an alternative, widely applicable approach that only uses the intrinsic features of the acquired DW-MRI data to track and correct motion to reliably reconstruct models of the renal diffusion signal. Unlike dynamic MRI techniques that make assumptions about the respiratory motion phases [3,17], we keep our technique generic and widely applicable by not making any specific assumptions about the type and source of motion.

Our proposed motion-robust spatially constrained parameter estimation (MOSCOPE) technique for kidney diffusion-weighted MRI is based on robust state estimation [1] for dynamic motion modeling, and 3D slice-to-volume image registration, which has been used in several challenging body imaging applications [5,6,10,12,13,18]. This approach uses the image features of 2D diffusion-sensitized slices which are the smallest packets of k-space data, each acquired in about 200 ms. This high sampling rate in renal DW-MRI allows effective estimation of physiological motion via a slice registration algorithm adapted from [19]. The estimated motion parameters are then applied to correct the position of each slice in 3D, which leads to scattered point cloud data, that is used in (1) spatially-constrained model fitting [15] for robust estimation of IVIM model parameters, and (2) weighted least squares estimation of diffusion tensor model parameters.

We evaluated the improvement in precision of parameter estimations using bootstrap-sampling on *in-vivo* DW-MRI datasets of 10 kidneys from 5 volunteers; and compared coefficient of variation percent (CV%) of the MOSCOPE parameter estimates to the CV% of the parameter estimates obtained from (1) the original DW-MRI data, and (2) rigid volume-to-volume registration of DW-MRI data. We also reconstructed diffusion tensor models in the kidney parenchyma and performed whole-kidney tractography. Our experimental results show that by estimating motion at the slice level, MOSCOPE allows better spatiotemporal resolution in motion correction and model reconstruction.

2   Methods

2.1   Renal DW-MRI Acquisition

Kidney DW-MRI involved free-breathing single-shot echo-planar imaging using the following parameters: repetition/echo time (TR/TE)=3300/91ms; matrix size=158×118; field of view=360×270 mm; slice thickness/gap $= 4$ mm/0 mm; 16 coronal slices; 10 b-values $= 0, 10, 30, 80, 120, 200, 400, 600, 800$ s/mm^2, 17 gradient directions; 10 $b = 0$ images; total acquisition time=10.7 min. This protocol allowed sequential acquisition of $N = 16 \times 9 \times 17 + 16 \times 10 \times 1 = 2608$ DW-MRI slices.

2.2   3D Motion Tracking and Correction of Sequentially Acquired Slices

We propose to track and estimate physiological motion (including respiratory motion) based on the information content of the sequential DW-MRI slice acquisitions. Given N DW-MRI slices, $\mathbf{y}_k$, and the associated d degree-of-freedom motion parameters $\mathbf{x}_k$ at each instant of slice acquisition, we formulate the dynamics of motion with a state space model:

$$\mathbf{x}_k = \mathbf{x}_{k-1} + \mathbf{w}_{k-1}; \quad \mathbf{y}_k = \mathbf{I}(\mathbf{x})_k + \mathbf{v}_k; \quad k = 1, ..., N; \tag{1}$$

where $\mathbf{w}_k$ and $\mathbf{v}_k$ are the process and measurement noise that represent the uncertainty in modeling the motion dynamics and the slice acquisitions, respectively. Given N $\mathbf{y}_k$s, we aim to estimate the motion states $\mathbf{x}_k$. The solution for motion tracking constitutes estimating the a posteriori probability density function $p(\mathbf{x}_k|\mathbf{y}_0, ...\mathbf{y}_k)$. For this purpose we use robust state estimation [1] as it was recently used in the algorithm proposed in [19]. To this end, we solve the state estimation problem through 3D slice-to-volume image registration, where we assume a moving window of size $2h + 1$, that maps the set of slices $\mathbf{y}_k = \mathbf{y}_{k-h}, ..., \mathbf{y}_{k+h}$ to a reference volume. The window size controls the bias-variance trade-off in the estimation of the motion parameters.

For sequential slice registration-based motion tracking, the first b=$0s/mm^2$ (B0) image is used as the initial reference volume. Then, an average B0 image is reconstructed after one iteration of slice motion correction. This averaged B0 image is used as reference to register next set of b values, i.e. b=$10s/mm^2$ images, followed by reconstruction of an average diffusion-sensitized image (B10) from b=$10s/mm^2$ images. The output (B10) image is used as the reference for the reconstruction of the next set of b value images, and the process repeats for all b-values; in this case finishing at b=$800s/mm^2$. At the end, we have reconstructed average reference images for all the b values, which were used as reference images to estimate motion parameters for all DW-MRI slices over time using the proposed sequential slice registration technique. After motion-compensation, we estimate both IVIM and diffusion tensor model parameters in cortex and medulla compartments of kidney parenchyma.

2.3   Spatially Constrained IVIM Parameter Estimation

The intravoxel incoherent motion (IVIM) model [16] represents the two-component isotropic diffusion signal decay with a bi-exponential function that has two decay rate parameters, one for the slow (D) and one for the fast diffusion (D*) and a parameter representing the fraction of fast diffusion (f):

$$S_i = S_0(f.e^{b_i(D+D^*)} + (1-f)e^{b_iD})\tag{2}$$

at b-value b_i, where $i \in \{1, 2, ..10\}$ is the index of b-value and S_0 is the signal at b=$0s/mm^2$. The parameters $\theta = [S_0, D, D^*, f]$ at each voxel can be estimated by solving a maximum-likelihood (ML) estimation problem. In order to improve IVIM parameter estimation accuracy from low SNR abdominal DW-MRI signal, instead of solving the ML optimization for each voxel independently, we use the recently developed spatially constrained IVIM (SC-IVIM) model fitting technique, where a spatial homogeneity prior model [7, 15] is added into the formulation. The parameters of the spatially constrained IVIM model are estimated by maximizing the posterior distribution given by the product of likelihood and prior terms given by

$$p(S|\Theta)p(\Theta) \propto \prod_v p(S_v|\Theta_v) \prod_{v_p \sim v_q} p(\Theta_{v_p}, \Theta_{v_q})\tag{3}$$

where each spatial prior term is defined over a neighborhood around voxel v_p. This optimization problem can be formulated as a continuous Markov Random Fields problem where the spatial homogeneity prior is defined as the L1 norm of the difference between parameters of neighboring voxels. To efficiently estimate the model parameters, we used the "fusion bootstrap moves" solver [7].

2.4   Weighted Least Squares Diffusion Tensor Model Estimation

For diffusion tensor model estimation based on the Stejskal-Tanner equation:

$$S_i = \tilde{S}_0 e^{-bg_i^T Dg_i},\tag{4}$$

where S_0 and S_i are the intensity values of the b=0 image and the diffusion sensitized images, respectively. We compute this model through weighted least squares estimation based on the following formula:

$$f(\gamma) = \frac{1}{2}\sum_{i=1}^n \omega_i^2 \alpha_i^2 \left(\ln\left(\frac{S_i}{\tilde{S}_0}\right) - \sum_{j=1}^6 M_{i,j}\gamma_j\right)^2,\tag{5}$$

in which $\gamma = [D_{xx}, D_{xy}, D_{xz}, D_{yy}, D_{yz}, D_{zz}]$ is a vector of 6 diffusion tensor model parameters; $M_{i,j}$ is the $n \times 6$ diffusion tensor design matrix based on the transformed gradient directions (g_i's) and the b values; and the weights ω_i's are defined by a kernel function based on the distances r_i's of n scattered points within the range of the kernel to the center of the ith voxel:

$$w_i = \frac{1}{\sigma\sqrt{2\pi}}e^{-\frac{1}{2}(\frac{r_i}{\sigma})^2} \tag{6}$$

The second set of weights (α_i) are set to S_i as suggested in [22], to account for the nonlinearity of the diffusion tensor model. Note that the g_i's in $\mathrm{M}_{i,j}$ are the gradient directions corrected by the motion parameters estimated for each slice; i.e. $g_i = \mathrm{R}_k g_{0i}$, where g_{0i} is the ith predefined gradient direction in the scanner coordinates, and R_k is the rotation matrix corresponding to the transformation $\mathbf{x}_k$ calculated for slice k by the motion estimator in Sect. 2.2. Based on the estimated tensor model for all voxels, we perform whole kidney tractography using a locally deterministic step tractography with 8 tract seeds and 5 steps per voxel, minimum fractional anisotropy threshold of 0.1, and a stopping mask on the entire kidney parenchyma.

3   Results

We tested the performance of MOSCOPE in DW-MRI of 10 kidneys from 5 healthy volunteers scanned on a 3 T scanner (Skyra, Siemens Medical Solutions, Erlangen, Germany). We assumed a 3D, 6 degree-of-freedom rigid motion model for each slice, and h was set to 2. We approximated the non-rigid motion as a combination of local rigid motion models around each kidney.

Using the proposed motion estimation technique, we measured three rotation and three translation parameters of each slice. Figure 1 shows the motion parameters calculated by the motion tracking algorithm (Sect. 2.2) plotted against

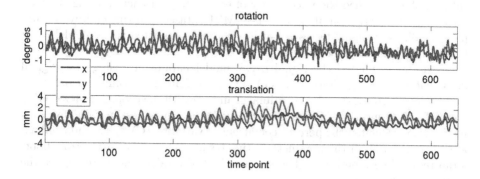

Fig. 1. The rotation (top) and translation (bottom) parameters of estimated physiological motion by the robust state space model estimation in Sect. 2.2. The x-axis points correspond to the sequentially acquired slices. The bottom red and green lines show periodic translation in the z (head-to-foot) and y (back-to-front) directions consistent in magnitude and frequency with respiratory motion of the diaphragm. Translation in the x (left-to-right) direction, shown by the blue line, was limited to a small drift. (Color figure online)

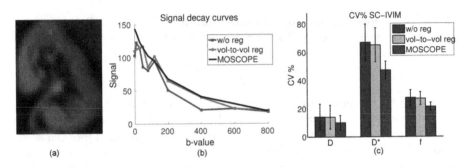

Fig. 2. (a) Motion-corrected b = 0 image using MOSCOPE method, (b) Signal decay curves of a voxel (red square in the first image) compared for without registration (w/o reg), with volume-to-volume registration (vol-to-vol reg), and MOSCOPE methods. MOSCOPE led to the most effective motion correction and model estimation. (c) Bar plot of CV% of multiple bootstrap parameter estimates are shown using the SC-IVIM model for w/o reg, vol-to-vol reg, and MOSCOPE methods. The reduction in CV% using the MOSCOPE method was statistically significant (paired student t-test at α threshold of 0.01) compared to w/o reg and vol-to-vol reg methods for all 3 parameters. (Color figure online)

time in seconds for one of the subjects. It is observed that the registration-based motion tracking algorithm accurately estimated large respiratory motion in two directions (z: head-to-foot, y:back-to-front), while found very small translational motion in the left-to-right direction. The magnitude and frequency of the translation in z and y directions was consistent with the expected respiratory motion.

Regions of kidney parenchyma including medulla and cortex and excluding kidney pelvis were delineated on DW-MRI images of both kidneys of each subject. We quantified the uncertainty of estimating parameters using the wild bootstrap analysis [8] on all *in-vivo* DW-MRI datasets. To this end, we resampled the diffusion signal for each b-value from the estimated signal model using the bootstrap resampling strategy.

Next, we estimated the signal decay model parameters using (1) original data, without registration (w/o reg); (2) with volume-to-volume registration (vol-to-vol reg) to the b = $0 s/mm^2$ image; and (3) with the proposed MOSCOPE method. As a measure of the uncertainty of parameter estimation, for each method we calculated the percent coefficient of variation (CV% = standard deviation/mean ×100) of the parameter estimates at each voxel over multiple bootstrap resampling repetitions. The smaller the CV% value, the more precise the parameter estimation.

Results are plotted in Fig. 2; where a motion-corrected b=0 image is shown in (a), and (b) compares the signal decay curves of a voxel of original signal without (w/o) motion compensation (blue), motion compensation with volume-to-volume registration (red) and MOSCOPE in black. MOSCOPE achieved a smooth exponential decaying signal while the other two decay curves had jumps. Also Fig. 2(c) shows that MOSCOPE led to the lowest (best) CV% values for all three parameters of the IVIM model, indicating the lowest uncertainties in parameter estimation. Using MOSCOPE the CV% of D, f, and D* parameters were reduced by 4%, 20%, and 7%, respectively compared to the CV% of w/o motion compensation method. The reduction in CV% using MOSCOPE was statistically significant (paired student t-test at α threshold of 0.01; $p < 0.01$) compared to the w/o reg and vol-to-vol reg methods for all 3 parameters.

The parameter maps of the IVIM model for kidney parenchyma regions in one of the experiments is shown in Fig. 3.

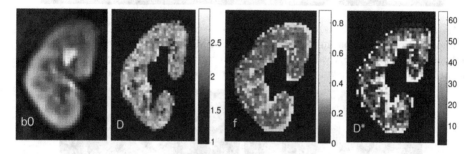

Fig. 3. The b=0 image, and parameter maps of D, D* and f parameters of the SC-IVIM model. Medulla has more restricted diffusion (D) than cortex. Medulla regions have high f (perfusion fraction) value compared to nearby cortex regions. Cortex regions with high vascularity also show high f values.

We compared the fractional anisotropy (FA) maps and values obtained from diffusion tensor models computed using (a) w/o registration, (b) vol-to-vol registration, and (c) MOSCOPE. Table 1 reports and compares mean FA values in the medulla and cortex for the three methods, and Fig. 4 shows the FA maps in one of the kidneys. Overall, MOSCOPE achieved the highest FA values in the medulla, while the other two methods resulted in reduced FA values, artifacts, and blurrier FA maps. Figure 5 shows tractography results in the left and right kidneys of a subject, without registration in (a) and with MOSCOPE in (b).

Table 1. The results showed that medulla has higher anisotropy with higher FA values compared to the cortex. The MOSCOPE method resulted in a significantly higher difference in the FA values (using paired student t-test) of medulla and cortex compared to without registration (w/o reg) and volume-to-volume registration (vol-to-vol reg).

	w/o reg	vol-to-vol reg	MOSCOPE
FA medulla	0.28 ± 0.05	0.26 ± 0.05	0.30 ± 0.04
FA cortex	0.21 ± 0.02	0.21 ± 0.02	0.20 ± 0.01

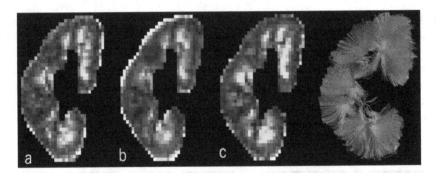

Fig. 4. FA maps from (a) w/o reg. (b) with vol-to-vol reg. and (c) MOSCOPE are compared. Motion robust parameter estimation with MOSCOPE resulted in the sharpest FA maps with highest FA values in the medulla regions. Tractography results obtained from MOSCOPE are shown on the right, where tracts are color coded by direction.

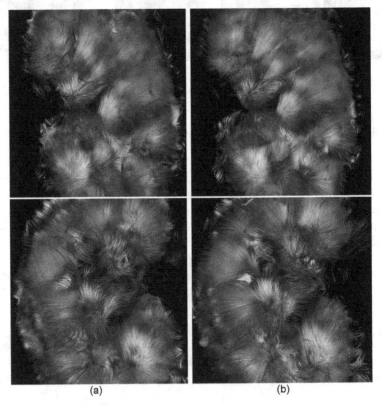

(a)   (b)

Fig. 5. Tractography based on the diffusion tensor model in the left and right kidneys of a subject, (a) without registration; and (b) with MOSCOPE. While we achieved robust diffusion tensor model fitting through constrained weighted least squares estimation (Sect. 2.4), the improvement achieved through motion correction using MOSCOPE is still observed in the images in (b) compared to (a). The tracts corresponding to the tubules in medulla region of the kidney are sharper in (b) compared to (a).

4   Conclusion

In this paper we introduced MOSCOPE for motion-compensated model estimation in renal DW-MRI. The technique has three main components: (1) we adapted an approach based on robust state estimation [1], which was recently utilized to solve slice-based motion estimation [19], to track physiological motion (including respiratory motion); (2) we used motion compensated data to achieve improved IVIM model estimation using a spatially constrained method; and (3) we used weighted least squares to estimate diffusion tensor model and perform tractography from motion-compensated data. For practical reasons (due to limited SNR and large slice thickness), we assumed rigid slice-level motion and used a non-causal model for motion tracking. Our formulation, however, is generic and can be used with deformable motion models, or in a causal form for prospective motion tracking. With better MR hardware and pulse sequences leading to improved SNR and higher resolution, more complex motion models may further improve the results, and more efficient implementations on powerful processing units may allow prospective motion tracking and near real-time reconstruction. In-vivo experiments with bootstrap sampling showed that the proposed method significantly reduced the uncertainty of parameter estimation. Precise quantitative diffusion-weighted imaging has the potential to be reliably used in clinic to identify renal pathologies where kidney function is compromised [2,9,11,21]. Our motion-compensated DW-MRI framework can also be used with other signal decay models of kidneys such as combined diffusion tensor-IVIM model [20] or 3-compartment signal decay model [24].

Acknowledgements. This work was supported in part by a Career Development Award from the Crohn's and Colitis Foundation to S. Kurugol, and in part by the National Institutes of Health (NIH) grants R01 DK100404, R01 EB018988, and R01 EB019483.

References

1. Agamennoni, G., Nieto, J.I., Nebot, E.M.: Approximate inference in state-space models with heavy-tailed noise. IEEE Trans. Signal Process. **60**(10), 5024–5037 (2012)
2. Bane, O., Wagner, M., Zhang, J.L., Dyvorne, H.A., Orton, M., et al.: Assessment of renal function using intravoxel incoherent motion diffusion-weighted imaging and dynamic contrast-enhanced MRI. J. Magn. Reson. Imaging **44**(2), 317–326 (2016)
3. Buerger, C., Clough, R.E., King, A.P., Schaeffter, T., Prieto, C.: Nonrigid motion modeling of the liver from 3-D undersampled self-gated golden-radial phase encoded MRI. IEEE Trans. Med. Imaging **31**(3), 805–815 (2012)
4. Eisenberger, U., Binser, T., Thoeny, H.C., Boesch, C., Frey, F.J., et al.: Living renal allograft transplantation: diffusion-weighted MR imaging in longitudinal follow-up of the donated and the remaining kidney. Radiology **270**(3), 800–808 (2013)
5. Fei, B., Duerk, J.L., Boll, D.T., et al.: Slice-to-volume registration and its potential application to interventional MRI-guided radio-frequency thermal ablation of prostate cancer. IEEE Trans. Med. Imaging **22**(4), 515–525 (2003)

6. Ferrante, E., Paragios, N.: Slice-to-volume medical image registration: A survey. Med. Image Anal. **39**, 101–123 (2017)

7. Freiman, M., Perez-Rossello, J.M., Callahan, M.J., Voss, S.D., et al.: Reliable estimation of incoherent motion parametric maps from diffusion-weighted MRI using fusion bootstrap moves. Med. Image Anal. **17**(3), 325–336 (2013)

8. Freiman, M., Voss, S.D., Mulkern, R.V., Perez-Rossello, J.M., Warfield, S.K.: Quantitative body DW-MRI biomarkers uncertainty estimation using unscented wild-bootstrap. In: Fichtinger, G., Martel, A., Peters, T. (eds.) MICCAI 2011. LNCS, vol. 6892, pp. 74–81. Springer, Heidelberg (2011). doi:10.1007/978-3-642-23629-7_10

9. Gaudiano, C., Clementi, V., Busato, F., Corcioni, B., Orrei, M.G., Ferramosca, E., et al.: Diffusion tensor imaging and tractography of the kidneys: assessment of chronic parenchymal diseases. Eur. Radiol. **23**(6), 1678–1685 (2013)

10. Gholipour, A., Estroff, J.A., Warfield, S.K.: Robust super-resolution volume reconstruction from slice acquisitions: application to fetal brain MRI. IEEE Trans. Med. Imaging **29**(10), 1739–1758 (2010)

11. Hueper, K., Khalifa, A., et al.: Diffusion-weighted imaging and diffusion tensor imaging detect delayed graft function and correlate with allograft fibrosis in patients early after kidney transplantation. J. Magn. Reson. Imaging **44**(1), 112–121 (2016)

12. Kainz, B., Steinberger, M., Wein, W., et al.: Fast volume reconstruction from motion corrupted stacks of 2D slices. IEEE Trans. Med. Imaging **34**(9), 1901–1913 (2015)

13. Kuklisova-Murgasova, M., Quaghebeur, G., Rutherford, M.A., Hajnal, J.V., Schnabel, J.A.: Reconstruction of fetal brain MRI with intensity matching and complete outlier removal. Med. Image Anal. **16**(8), 1550–1564 (2012)

14. Kurugol, S., Freiman, M., Afacan, O., Domachevsky, L., Perez-Rossello, J.M., Callahan, M.J., Warfield, S.K.: Motion-robust parameter estimation in abdominal diffusion-weighted MRI by simultaneous image registration and model estimation. Med. Image Anal. **39**, 124–132 (2017)

15. Kurugol, S., Freiman, M., Afacan, O., et al.: Spatially-constrained probability distribution model of incoherent motion for abdominal diffusion weighted MRI. Med. Image Anal. **32**, 173–183 (2016)

16. Le Bihan, D., Breton, E., Lallemand, D., Aubin, M., Vignaud, J., Laval-Jeantet, M.: Separation of diffusion and perfusion in intravoxel incoherent motion MR imaging. Radiology **168**(2), 497–505 (1988)

17. Lin, W., Guo, J., Rosen, M.A., Song, H.K.: Respiratory motion-compensated radial dynamic contrast-enhanced (DCE)-MRI of chest and abdominal lesions. Magn. Reson. Med. **60**(5), 1135–1146 (2008)

18. Marami, B., Salehi, S.S.M., Afacan, O., Scherrer, B., Rollins, C.K., Yang, E., Estroff, J.A., Warfield, S.K., Gholipour, A.: Temporal slice registration and robust diffusion-tensor reconstruction for improved fetal brain structural connectivity analysis. NeuroImage **156**(1), 475–488 (2017)

19. Marami, B., Scherrer, B., Afacan, O., Erem, B., Warfield, S.K., Gholipour, A.: Motion-robust diffusion-weighted brain MRI reconstruction through slice-level registration-based motion tracking. IEEE Trans. Med. Imaging **35**(10), 2258–2269 (2016)

20. Notohamiprodjo, M., Chandarana, H., et al.: Combined intravoxel incoherent motion and diffusion tensor imaging of renal diffusion and flow anisotropy. Magn. Reson. Med. **73**(4), 1526–1532 (2014)

21. Paudyal, B., Paudyal, P., Tsushima, Y., Oriuchi, N., Amanuma, M., Miyazaki, M., et al.: The role of the ADC value in the characterisation of renal carcinoma by diffusion-weighted MRI. Br. J. Radiol. **83**(988), 336–343 (2010)
22. Salvador, R., Peña, A., Menon, D.K., Carpenter, T.A., Pickard, J.D., Bullmore, E.T.: Formal characterization and extension of the linearized diffusion tensor model. Hum. Brain Mapp. **24**(2), 144–155 (2005)
23. Seif, M., Lu, H., Boesch, C., Reyes, M., Vermathen, P.: Image registration for triggered and non-triggered DTI of the human kidney: Reduced variability of diffusion parameter estimation. J. Magn. Reson. Imaging **41**(5), 1228–1235 (2015)
24. Van Baalen, S., Leemans, A., Dik, P., Lilien, M.R., Ten Haken, B., Froeling, M.: Intravoxel incoherent motion modeling in the kidneys: Comparison of mono-, bi- and triexponential fit. J. Magn. Reson. Imaging **46**(1), 228–239 (2017)

Semi-automatic Cardiac and Respiratory Gated MRI for Cardiac Assessment During Exercise

Bram Ruijsink[1,2](✉), Esther Puyol-Antón[1], Muhammad Usman[1,3],
Joshua van Amerom[1], Phuoc Duong[1,2], Mari Nieves Velasco Forte[1,2],
Kuberan Pushparajah[1,2], Alessandra Frigiola[1,2], David A. Nordsletten[1],
Andrew P. King[1], and Reza Razavi[1,2]

[1] Division of Imaging Sciences and Biomedical Engineering,
King's College London, London, UK
jacobus.ruijsink@kcl.ac.uk
[2] Guy's and St Thomas' Hospital NHS Foundation Trust, London, UK
[3] Department of Computer Science, University College London, London, UK

Abstract. Imaging of the heart during exercise can improve detection and treatment of heart diseases but is challenging using current clinically applied cardiac MRI (cMRI) techniques. Real-time (RT) imaging strategies have recently been proposed for exercise cMRI, but respiratory motion and unreliable cardiac gating introduce significant errors in quantification of cardiac function. Self-navigated cMRI sequences are currently not routinely available in a clinical environment. We aim to establish a method for cardiac and respiratory gated cine exercise cMRI that can be applied in a clinical cMRI setting. We developed a retrospective, image-based cardiac and respiratory gating and reconstruction framework based on widely available highly accelerated dynamic imaging. From the acquired dynamic images, respiratory motion was estimated using manifold learning. Cardiac periodicity was obtained by identifying local maxima in the temporal frequency spectrum of the spatial means of the images. We then binned the dynamic images in respiratory and cardiac phases and subsequently registered and averaged them to reconstruct a respiratory and cardiac gated cine stack. We evaluated our method in healthy volunteers and patients with heart diseases and demonstrate good agreement with existing RT acquisitions (R = .82). We show that our reconstruction pipeline yields better image quality and has lower inter- and intra-observer variability compared to RT imaging. Subsequently, we demonstrate that our method is able to detect a pathological response to exercise in patients with heart diseases, illustrating its potential benefit in cardiac diagnostic and prognostic assessment.

Keywords: Exercise MRI · Cardiac imaging · Image-based motion correction · Manifold learning

1 Introduction

Assessment of cardiac volumes, function and wall motion using cardiac Magnetic Resonance Imaging (cMRI) during physiological stress (exercise) has a

© Springer International Publishing AG 2017
M.J. Cardoso et al. (Eds.): CMMI/RAMBO/SWITCH 2017, LNCS 10555, pp. 86–95, 2017.
DOI: 10.1007/978-3-319-67564-0_9

great potential to improve early diagnosis, treatment evaluation and prognostic stratification in patients with heart disease [2, 10]. Unfortunately, visualising the heart during exercise is challenging using routine clinical cMRI as bodily movements and the inability to breath hold severely corrupt quality of the images (see Fig. 3a).

In an attempt to enable imaging during exercise, several clinical research groups have proposed the use of non-gated real-time (RT) MRI sequences [10, 13]. These highly accelerated imaging techniques sacrifice spatial resolution and signal-to-noise ratio (SNR) compared to breath held, ECG gated cine cMRI (conventional cine) to produce images that are not corrupted by motion, see example in Fig. 3b. Although the resulting images allow assessment of cardiac function during exercise, through-plane motion of the heart during respiration and bodily movements during exercise lead to significant errors and variability in quantification of cardiac volumes and function [3] and complicate the assessment of wall motion abnormalities. Furthermore, due to the presence of multiple heart beats in one acquisition inter- and intra-observer variability in choice for target images for assessment of cardiac volumes are likely to add further errors, limiting the potential use of RT imaging for clinical application.

To account for respiratory motion during free-breathing cMRI, a navigator echo is typically added to cMRI sequences [15]. However, this method reduces temporal resolution of dynamic imaging, making it unsuitable for use during exercise. Several self-navigating (SG) sequences have recently been developed that account for respiratory and cardiac motion during cMRI. In SG, target motion is estimated directly from the acquired data. As a result, most SG techniques do not increase scan-time or reduce temporal resolution. SG techniques can be divided in image-based, k-space based, and model-based approaches. Image-based SG relies on registration of high quality dynamic images based on motion signals derived from lower temporal or spatial dimensional images reconstructed from the same dataset [11, 12, 14, 17]. K-space based methods derive the respiratory signal from central k-space lines [4, 5, 9]. Finally, model-based approaches have been proposed for motion detection in cMRI. An example of such an approach is described by Yoon et al. [18], who use a low-rank method that separates the background of the image mathematically from the dynamic portions. Although the above described SG techniques have great potential for imaging during exercise, the proposed methods rely on complex k-space trajectories, such as radial [11, 12] or golden angle radial [5, 14, 17] acquisition schemes, and computer intensive reconstruction frameworks. Unfortunately, such techniques are currently not widely available in a clinical cMRI setting, limiting their use for routine clinical exercise cMRI. Hansen et al. proposed a method for image-based respiratory gating at rest, based on a real-time cMRI sequence that is standardly available on commercial MRI systems [8]. However, this technique uses ECG waveforms for cardiac gating; a strategy that is not feasible for imaging during exercise as ECG signals are significantly disturbed due to bodily motion.

In this work, we develop and evaluate a semi-automatic framework for reconstruction of cardiac and respiratory gated cine cMRI (exGated cine) that allows for assessment of cardiac volumes, function and wall motion during strenuous physical exercise. In order to maximise application of our technique in clinical cMRI settings, we aimed for a method with minimal user interaction that can be flexibly applied on all imaging platforms without the need for advanced sequence programming or the use of intensive computing power. We show that our technique, based on a widely available real-time imaging sequence, is able to reconstruct gated cine images with improved image quality and lower inter-and intra-observer variability than non-gated RT imaging. Furthermore, we demonstrate that our method allows detection of a pathological cardiac response to exercise in patients with a heart disease.

2   Methods

We propose a strategy that involves (i) acquisition of highly accelerated dynamic (real-time) MRI using widely available acceleration techniques followed by (ii) image-based cardiac synchronisation, (iii) respiratory gating and (iv) motion correction and reconstruction of a 24–30 phase cardiac cine image stack. We evaluated our method in 10 healthy volunteers and 10 patients with congenital heart diseases (CHD) and exercise intolerance. Dynamic imaging datasets were acquired at moderate and high intensity, supine bicycle ergometer exercise corresponding to a heart rate (HR) of $\sim$100–110 beats per minute (bpm) and $\sim$135–150 bpm, respectively. As routinely used clinical cine cMRI (conventional cine) is not feasible during exercise, we compared exGated cine with a previously validated, non-gated real-time imaging protocol (non-gated RT) that uses manual selection of respiratory state using a dedicated cardiac analysis software package (RightVol, KU Leuven) [10]. We assessed agreement between the two methods using Pearson's correlation, assessed inter- and intra-observer variability with Bland Altman plots and tested for difference in variance between the two methods using the F-ratio. Image quality was rated using a 5-point Image Quality Score (IQS; 1 = unsuitable for diagnostic use, 5 = similar to conventional cine imaging at rest) by two blinded imaging-cardiologist. Lastly, we compared systolic function between healthy volunteers and patients with CHD during exercise using a repeated measures ANOVA with exercise intensity as the within-subject effect. Values are expressed as means $\pm$ SD. $p < .05$ was considered statistically significant. The main novelty of the proposed method lies in the clinical applicability of our semi-automatic, image-based reconstruction framework that creates respiratory and cardiac gated cine images of the heart during exercise without the need for intensive computing power or advanced cMRI pulse-sequences. The proposed framework is illustrated in Fig. 1. Our pipeline was implemented in MATLAB R2015b (MathWorks, Natick, USA) utilizing the signal processing, image processing and statistics toolboxes. This study has been approved by our regional ethics board (REC: 15/LO/522, Bloomsbury London,UK) and informed consent was obtained from all participants.

2.1 Highly Accelerated Dynamic MRI

Our method relies on high temporal resolution (~35 ms/frame) dynamic imaging, using acceleration techniques that are currently available on all commercially available MRI scanners, without the need of advanced user settings. In this study, images were acquired on a 1.5T MRI scanner (Ingenia, Philips Medical, Best, The Netherlands). Steady-state free precession imaging was performed without cardiac gating. 80–100 consecutive frames were acquired over 14 slices with a thickness of 8 mm in a short axis orientation. Imaging parameters were: field of view, 300×260 mm (approx.); flip angle 50°; SENSE factor 3 (Cartesian k-space undersampling); partial Fourier factor 0.5, repetition time 1.8 ms; echo time 0.9 ms and reconstruction-matrix, 128×112, resulting in a reconstructed voxel size, $2.3 \times 2.3 \times 8$ ms and a frame rate of ~35 ms. After acquisition, a region of interest around the heart (cROI) and a centre point for the LV were manually selected on an average of all images to facilitate the reconstruction process. This is the only manual step of our pipeline.

exGated cine MRI pipeline

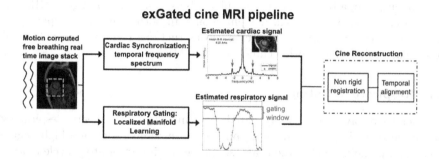

Fig. 1. Overview of the proposed framework for cardiac and respiratory gated MRI during exercise.

2.2 Cardiac Synchronization

ECG signals, routinely used for cardiac gating in cMRI, are significantly distorted during physical exercise. However, the high temporal resolution of our acquisition allows for direct estimation of the cardiac periodicity from the images, as was previously demonstrated by van Amerom et al. [1]. In order to obtain cardiac gating, we estimated the cardiac periodicity during exercise by transforming the images to the frequency domain and taking the spatial mean of the cROI. Before Fourier transformation the signal was interpolated to a resolution of 0.03 bpm (0.05 mHz) by zero-padding in the time domain. The local maxima in the frequency spectrum within the range of fundamental frequencies (0.8–2.8 Hz) were identified and used to calculate cardiac periodicity (see Fig. 2a). Subsequently, each frame was assigned to an associated cardiac phase bin based

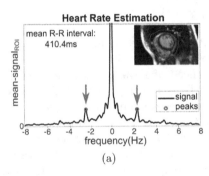
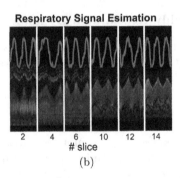

Fig. 2. (a) Range of fundamental frequencies (1.8–2.7 Hz) of the temporal frequency domain, estimated cardiac rate on the ROI appeared as the maxima (red arrows). (b) Estimated respiratory signal (red line) overlay to a spatio-temporal intensity profile through diaphragm. (Color figure online)

on the cardiac time interval. For HRs <130 bpm, the cardiac time interval was divided in 30 equally spaced cardiac phase bins, whereas for higher HRs the frames were divided over 24 cardiac phase bins. In both cases, the temporal resolution (in cardiac phases) of the cine reconstructions comply with guidelines for cine acquisitions in routine clinical cardiac MRI [6].

2.3   Respiratory Gating

In order to resolve high quality gated cine imaging of the heart, respiratory motion needs to be corrected. As respiratory excursions result in a high degree of through-plane motion of the heart, simply averaging respiratory cycle motion throughout the acquisition would lead to significant blurring of the reconstructed images. This also deviates from the current standard of end-expiratory assessment of cardiac volumes. We therefore applied Laplacian Eigenmaps, a Manifold Learning (ML) technique, in order to automatically estimate the respiratory motion in each slice in the imaging stack based on image intensity [17]. ML projects a higher dimensional manifold (e.g., an image of large dimensions) to a corresponding low dimensional representation. Previous work has shown that this technique is be able to accurately estimate a 1D representation of respiratory motion from dynamic cardiac imaging at rest [17]. As the ML estimated respiratory signal may have cardiac component due to high temporal resolution of real-time images, we filtered this signal in the frequency range of 0.1–0.5 Hz in order to retain the respiratory component. Subsequently a predefined respiratory gating window was used to select the images at end-expiration (20% of respiratory movement from maximal expiration) for further reconstruction. This gating window is equivalent to a ~6–8 mm gating window using a respiratory navigator echo. Figure 2b shows an example of the ML estimated respiratory signal overlaid on a spatio-temporal intensity profile through diaphragm.

Conventional cine MRI   **non-gated RT imaging**   **exGated cine MRI**

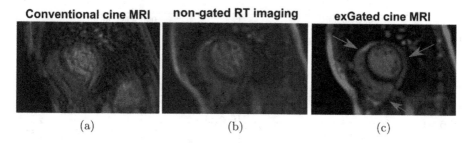

(a)   (b)   (c)

Fig. 3. Cardiac reconstructed MRI images: (a) conventional cine MRI, (b) non-gated RT MRI [10], (c) proposed approach - exGated cine MRI. Arrows denote better delineation of pericardium fat and RV wall of the proposed method.

2.4   Cine Reconstruction

After cardiac and respiratory gating, the most representative image within each cardiac phase bin was selected by computing the mean-square error between all image pairs in that bin. The image with lowest error with respect to all other images was selected as the reference image. Subsequently, a Demons non-rigid registration algorithm [16] was used to estimate the set of displacement fields that aligns each image to this reference image. All images were registered and averaged to form a unique image per bin, hereby improving SNR. In order to assure temporal alignment of the cardiac phases between all slices, we segmented the LV blood pool using an automatic segmentation algorithm based on Otsu's method that was guided by the cROI and LV centre point. The smallest segmentation of each slice was selected as the end-systolic frame. Based on this reference frame all slices were temporally aligned. Finally, a rigid body in-plane image registration was performed to register the position of the heart over time to reduce inter-frame exercise motion, facilitating the interpretation of ventricular contraction and wall motion abnormalities.

3   Experiments and Results

All datasets were successfully reconstructed to exGated cine stacks that allowed volumetric analysis. There was good agreement in ventricular stroke volume (SV) between exGated cine and non-gated RT imaging ($R = 0.82$). Bland Altman analysis of the two methods and their respective inter- and intra-observer agreement are shown in Figs. 4 and 5. The inter- and intra-observer variance of SV was significantly lower in exGated cine compared to RT imaging (intra-observer: $F_{(29,29)} = 2.75$, $p < .01$ and inter-observer: $F_{(29,29)} = 3.01$, $p < .01$). The IQS was $1.1 \pm .3$ for conventional cine, $3.1 \pm .6$ for non-gated RT and $3.9 \pm .5$ for exGated cine (see Fig. 6). Figure 3 shows an example of conventional cine, non-gated RT MRI and our gated cine approach, with good delineation of pericardial fat and RV-wall obtained by our proposed method. Lastly, we show that

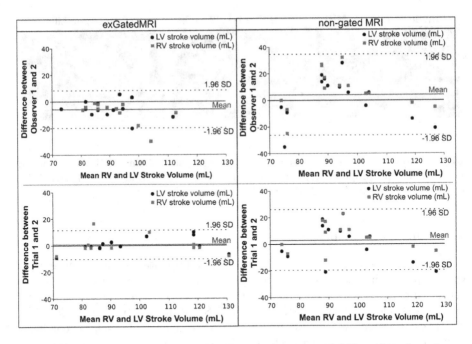

Fig. 4. Bland Altman plots of inter- and intra-observer variability of stroke volume (mL) of the two methods. Note the smaller limits of agreement and variance in exGated Cine.

the increase in LV systolic function (measured by ejection fraction) was significantly lower in patients with congenital heart disease and exercise intolerance compared to healthy volunteers ($p < .01$ for both moderate and high exercise), see Table 1.

Table 1. Ejection Fraction during exercise for patients with complex congenital heart disease (CHD) and healthy volunteers using the exGated cine MRI.

LV ejection fraction (%)	Healthy Volunteers (n = 10)	Patients with complex CHD (n = 10)
Rest	62 ± 5	51 ± 8
Moderate[a]	68 ± 4	53 ± 6
High[a]	74 ± 6	55 ± 4

[a] represents $p < .05$.

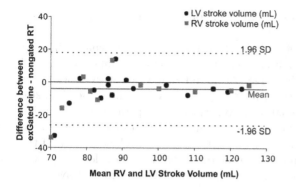

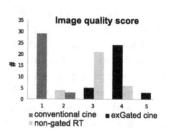

Fig. 5. Bland Altman plot of agreement in stroke volume (mL) between exGated cine and non-gated RT.

Fig. 6. Image quality score between conventional cine MRI (white bar), non-gate RT [10] (gray bar) and our proposed approach - exGated cine MRI (black bar).

4   Discussion

In this work, we present a reconstruction pipeline for cardiac and respiratory gated cine cMRI that allows for accurate assessment of cardiac function during strenuous physical exercise. Imaging of the heart during exercise has so far been restricted due to bodily motion and cardiac gating issues. However, its widely recognized potential for disease evaluation [2] appeals for exploration of techniques to enable exercise cMRI. No satisfying technique has yet been developed that allows widespread clinical implementation of exercise cMRI. RT imaging strategies suffer from significant errors in quantitative assessment due to respiratory motion [3]. Whereas SG strategies, recently developed and applied in MRI at rest [4,5,7,11,14,17], require custom-build cMRI pulse sequences and computationally expensive reconstruction schemes that are currently not available in most clinical cMRI environments.

We developed a method for exercise cMRI that can be directly applied in clinical practice. Our proposed reconstruction framework starts with the acquisition of a stack of highly accelerated dynamic images. This type of dynamic cMRI sequences is currently available on all commercial MRI scanners. Our proposed reconstruction framework starts with the acquisition of a stack of highly accelerated dynamic images. This type of dynamic cMRI sequences is currently available on all commercial MRI scanners. We exploit the temporal resolution of the acquired images for image-based estimation of cardiac and respiratory motion. By using image-based techniques, we avoid the use of raw image data and complex reconstruction techniques. In order to keep computational expenses low, we utilize dimensional reduction in our motion estimation techniques. As a result, our framework is able to reconstruct a cine stack of the heart in a clinically acceptable total reconstruction time of ~30–40 min using a standard laptop computer.

We used ML to estimate motion from the acquired stack of dynamic images. This method has previously been used in combination with dynamic imaging and shown to be both robust and fast [17]. We found that respiratory motion was accurately estimated with the ML using the entire image as input (see Fig. 2b). ML did also detect a cardiac signal. However, the cardiac periodicity estimation based on this signal proved to be not precise enough for cardiac gating, due to significant shifts in image intensities as a result of through-plane motion of the heart and surrounding fat. Estimation in the temporal frequency domain proved more accurate. However, we needed to introduce a cROI in order to avoid the detection of exercise motion.

We implemented our proposed reconstruction pipeline in our clinical cMRI facility and showed that the output of our reconstruction pipeline, exGated cine, is in acceptable agreement with non-gated RT imaging for SV. There is some variability in quantification of SV noted between the two methods. However, inter- and intra-observer variability of exGated cine was superior compared to non-gated RT imaging. These results most likely reflect the improved accuracy of exGated cine, as quantification errors introduced by respiratory motion in non-gated RT imaging are eliminated [3]. This improved repeatability in quantification of SV is an important gain of our technique, as it facilitates implementation of exercise cMRI in a clinical setting.

Finally, we demonstrated that our method was able to detect a clear pathophysiologic response to exercise in patients with CHD, expressed by the significantly lower increase in systolic function compared to healthy volunteers. This highlights the potential advantages of exercise cMRI for clinical cardiology. Our work is a preliminary step in the application of image processing techniques in the emerging field of exercise cMRI. We aim to improve our method further by implementing automatic segmentation techniques for detection and segmentation of the LV bloodpool. Some recently proposed self-gated cMRI sequences could have important potential for imaging during exercise. Unfortunately, translation of such techniques to clinical settings remains challenging. We hope that our work is an encouragement for development and implementation of these techniques for clinical exercise cMRI.

References

1. van Amerom, J., Lloyd, D., Price, A., Kuklisova Murgasova, M., Aljabar, P., Malik, S., Lohezic, M., Rutherford, M., Pushparajah, K., Razavi, R., et al.: Fetal cardiac cine imaging using highly accelerated dynamic MRI with retrospective motion correction and outlier rejection. Magn. Reson. Med. (2017)
2. Cahalin, L., Chase, P., Arena, R., Myers, J., Bensimhon, D., Peberdy, M., Ashley, E., West, E., Forman, D., Pinkstaff, S., et al.: A meta-analysis of the prognostic significance of cardiopulmonary exercise testing in patients with heart failure. Heart Fail. Rev. 18(1), 79–94 (2013)

3. Claessen, G., Claus, P., Delcroix, M., Bogaert, J., La Gerche, A., Heidbuchel, H.: Interaction between respiration and right versus left ventricular volumes at rest and during exercise: a real-time cardiac magnetic resonance study. Am. J. Physiol. Heart Circ. Physiol. **306**(6), H816–H824 (2014)

4. Crowe, M., Larson, A., Zhang, Q., Carr, J., White, R., Li, D., Simonetti, O.: Automated rectilinear self-gated cardiac cine imaging. Magn. Reson. Med. **52**(4), 782–788 (2004)

5. Feng, L., Axel, L., Chandarana, H., Block, K.T., Sodickson, D.K., Otazo, R.: XD-GRASP: golden-angle radial MRI with reconstruction of extra motion-state dimensions using compressed sensing. Magn. Reson. Med. **75**(2), 775–788 (2016)

6. Fratz, S., Chung, T., Greil, G., Samyn, M., Taylor, A., Buechel, E., Yoo, S.J., Powell, A.: Guidelines and protocols for cardiovascular magnetic resonance in children and adults with congenital heart disease: SCMR expert consensus group on congenital heart disease. J. Cardiovasc. Magn. Reson. **15**(1), 51 (2013)

7. Han, F., Zhou, Z., Han, E., Gao, Y., Nguyen, K.L., Finn, J., Hu, P.: Self-gated 4D multiphase, steady-state imaging with contrast enhancement (MUSIC) using rotating cartesian K-space (ROCK): validation in children with congenital heart disease. Magn. Reson. Med. (2016)

8. Hansen, M., Sørensen, T., Arai, A., Kellman, P.: Retrospective reconstruction of high temporal resolution cine images from real-time MRI using iterative motion correction. Magn. Reson. Med. **68**(3), 741–750 (2012)

9. Kim, W., Mun, C., Kim, D., Cho, Z.: Extraction of cardiac and respiratory motion cycles by use of projection data and its applications to nmr imaging. Magn. Reson. Med. **13**(1), 25–37 (1990)

10. La Gerche, A., Claessen, G., Van de Bruaene, A., Pattyn, N., Van Cleemput, J., Gewillig, M., Bogaert, J., Dymarkowski, S., Claus, P., Heidbuchel, H.: Cardiac MRI: a new gold standard for ventricular volume quantification during high-intensity exercise. Circ. Cardiovasc. Imaging **6**(2), 329–338 (2013)

11. Larson, A., White, R., Laub, G., McVeigh, E., Li, D., Simonetti, O.: Self-gated cardiac cine MRI. Magn. Reson. Med. **51**(1), 93–102 (2004)

12. Liu, C., Bammer, R., Kim, D.H., Moseley, M.: Self-navigated interleaved spiral (SNAILS): application to high-resolution diffusion tensor imaging. Magn. Reson. Med. **52**(6), 1388–1396 (2004)

13. Lurz, P., Muthurangu, V., Schievano, S., Nordmeyer, J., Bonhoeffer, P., Taylor, A., Hansen, M.: Feasibility and reproducibility of biventricular volumetric assessment of cardiac function during exercise using real-time radial k-t SENSE magnetic resonance imaging. J. Magn. Reson. Imaging **29**(5), 1062–1070 (2009)

14. Paul, J., Divkovic, E., Wundrak, S., Bernhardt, P., Rottbauer, W., Neumann, H., Rasche, V.: High-resolution respiratory self-gated golden angle cardiac MRI: comparison of self-gating methods in combination with k-t SPARSE SENSE. Magn. Reson. Med. **73**(1), 292–298 (2015)

15. Peters, D.C., Nezafat, R., Eggers, H., Stehning, C., Manning, W.J.: 2D free-breathing dual navigator-gated cardiac function validated against the 2D breath-hold acquisition. J. Magn. Reson. Imaging **28**(3), 773–777 (2008)

16. Thirion, J.P.: Image matching as a diffusion process: an analogy with Maxwell's demons. Med. Image Anal. **2**(3), 243–260 (1998)

17. Usman, M., Atkinson, D., Kolbitsch, C., Schaeffter, T., Prieto, C.: Manifold learning based ECG-free free-breathing cardiac CINE MRI. J. Magn. Reson. Imaging **41**(6), 1521–1527 (2015)

18. Yoon, H., Kim, K., Kim, D., Bresler, Y., Ye, J.: Motion adaptive patch-based low-rank approach for compressed sensing cardiac cine MRI. IEEE Trans. Med. Imaging **33**(11), 2069–2085 (2014)

CoronARe: A Coronary Artery Reconstruction Challenge

Serkan Çimen[1], Mathias Unberath[2(✉)], Alejandro Frangi[1], and Andreas Maier[2]

[1] Center for Computational Imaging and Simulation Technologies in Biomedicine,
The University of Sheffield, Sheffield, UK
[2] Pattern Recognition Lab, Friedrich-Alexander-Universität Erlangen-Nürnberg,
Erlangen, Germany
unberath@jhu.edu

Abstract. *CoronARe* ranks state-of-the-art methods in symbolic and tomographic coronary artery reconstruction from interventional C-arm rotational angiography. Specifically, we benchmark the performance of the methods using accurately pre-processed data, and study the effects of imperfect pre-processing conditions (segmentation and background subtraction errors). In this first iteration of the challenge, evaluation is performed in a controlled environment using digital phantom images, where accurate 3D ground truth is known.

Keywords: Angiography · 3D reconstruction · C-arm Cone-beam CT · Motion compensation

1 Introduction

Coronary artery disease (CAD) is a serious illness, which is responsible for approximately 20% of the deaths in Europe [1] and in the US [2]. Currently, clinical decision regarding the presence and the extent of CAD is taken by the help of several diagnostic and interventional medical imaging modalities. Among those, invasive (catheter-based) X-ray coronary angiography is still the most common choice for the assessment of CAD. Owing to its high spatial/temporal resolution and its availability, it is still considered as the gold standard in clinical decision making and therapy guidance [3].

The X-ray angiography systems evolved continuously since their first introduction almost five decades ago. However, X-ray coronary angiography is known to be fundamentally limited due to the projective 2D representation of the coronary artery trees with complex anatomy and motion. Misinterpretation of lesion lengths, eccentricity, angles of bifurcations and vessel tortuosity due to the 2D nature of the X-ray angiography could lead to over/under estimation of lesion severity and incorrect selection of stent size [4,5]. Methods computing reconstructions of coronary arteries from X-ray angiography aim to overcome this

---

S. Çimen and M. Unberath—Both authors contributed equally to this paper.

© Springer International Publishing AG 2017
M.J. Cardoso et al. (Eds.): CMMI/RAMBO/SWITCH 2017, LNCS 10555, pp. 96–104, 2017.
DOI: 10.1007/978-3-319-67564-0_10

shortcoming by providing 3D information of the coronary arteries. Due to the complexity of this task, the topic of reconstruction from X-ray coronary angiography remains as a challenging and active research area.

Public benchmarks contribute to drive forward this area as they allow for objective comparison of coronary artery reconstruction algorithms from rotational angiography. A previous effort, *CAVAREV* [6] laid the foundation for public benchmarks in this field but is limited to tomographic reconstruction algorithms.

Within the *CoronARe* challenge, we seek to continue the *CAVAREV* incentive by providing a public benchmark for both tomographic and symbolic reconstruction algorithms. In this first iteration of the challenge, we study current state-of-the-art reconstruction algorithms in a highly controlled setup on numerical phantom data, where accurate 3D and 2D data is available.

2   Materials and Methods

2.1   Scope and Specific Goals

The literature is divided into symbolic (i.e. model-based) and tomographic methods [7]. Symbolic reconstruction algorithms try to recover a binary representation of the topology of the arterial tree while tomographic reconstruction methods directly reconstruct the 3D volume of attenuation coefficients. Irrespective of their categorization as symbolic or tomographic, most currently known coronary artery reconstruction algorithms from rotational angiography rely on projection domain vessel segmentation or centerline extraction algorithms to either perform background suppression or obtain sparse data. Much work has considered automatic vessel segmentation [7–9] both in an analytic, model-based but also in a machine learning context. While results are promising when a static imaging geometry can be assumed (e.g. as in traditional angiography), satisfactory segmentation quality cannot yet be reliably achieved in rotational angiography because of substantial changes in vessel visibility in successive views due to overlap with high contrast structures, such as the spine.

Consequently, automatic segmentation algorithms inevitably lead to projection domain mis-segmentations and inconsistencies (which we will refer to as corruption) that have to be addressed during reconstruction. Within the challenge described here, we investigate how different methods cope with imperfect pre-processing of the projection images, i.e. errors in centerline segmentation and single-frame background subtraction based on vessel segmentation and inpainting. The setup of the challenge is described in greater detail in the remainder of this manuscript.

2.2   Data

Numerical Phantom. To create the controlled setup for benchmarking the reconstruction algorithms, we decided to use the 4D XCAT Phantom [10]. This phantom defines detailed and anatomically correct cardiac vasculature using non-uniform rational B-splines (NURBS). It also allows for the simulation of cardiac motion.

The left coronary artery (LCA) geometry of the XCAT phantom is used to generate the projection data for both symbolic and tomographic reconstruction parts of this challenge. A sequence of 133 NURBS descriptions of the LCA is simulated for the whole acquisition duration, where we set the heart rate to 80 beats per minute.

For the symbolic reconstruction, 3D ground truth is obtained by sampling the spline defining the centerlines at regular arc length intervals of 0.3 mm. For each projection in the sequence, the 3D spline is projected onto the corresponding image plane. Similar to 3D, points defining the uncorrupted centerline segmentations are sampled from these splines at regular arc length intervals of 2.0 mm.

In addition, the sequence of NURBS files are voxelized with an isotropic image spacing of 0.3 mm, and the values of the voxels corresponding to artery locations set to one, whereas remaining voxels are set to zero. A subvolume of size $512 \times 512 \times 360$ centered at the barycenter of the 3D ground truth points of the end-diastolic phase defines the ground truth for each time step in the sequence. The CT Projector [10] is used to simulate the projection images, which is capable of computing the sum of attenuation values analytically from NURBS definitions given the imaging geometry.

Imaging Geometry. The 4D numerical phantom is forward projected using the geometric calibration of a real scanner taken from *CAVAREV* [6] describing a standard rotational angiography protocol. In particular, 133 images are acquired during a single 5.3 s sweep on a circular source trajectory covering 200°. The projection images have a size of 960×960 pixels in horizontal and vertical direction, respectively, with an isotropic size of 0.32 mm. The source-to-isocenter and source-to-detector distances nominally are 800 mm and 1200 mm, respectively.

Artificial Corruption: Imperfect Preprocessing. Within this challenge, corruption of the acquisition will be random but with increasing severity. Particularly, for both the symbolic and tomographic data sets we use the uncorrupted acquisitions as the baseline and add excessive structure such that the corruption amounts to 10%, 20%, and 30% of the true information [11].

Symbolic Reconstruction. It is well known that the reconstruction problem in rotational angiography is ill-posed due to high frequency cardiac motion. Symbolic reconstruction algorithms exploit sparsity of the vessel centerlines to overcome this challenge suggesting that reconstruction results heavily depend on the quality of the centerlines.

To realistically simulate vessel extraction errors, points were sampled from random curves, and added to the true segmentation points following [11]. Specifically, random trajectories of particles were generated using Brownian motion, and smoothed by fitting cubic Hermite splines. The points corresponding to the vessel extraction errors were sampled from these splines at 2.0 mm, which is the same rate used for generating the true centerline segmentation.

Tomographic Reconstruction. Background subtraction or -suppression proved highly beneficial for reconstruction quality when considering both analytic and algebraic reconstruction algorithms [7], as it promotes sparsity and corrects for truncation [12]. This preprocessing step usually relies on binary masks of the target vessels to identify the contrasted lumen and, subsequently, virtually remove the background.

We simulate errors in the suppression process by generating a corruption image for each projection in the sequence, and adding it to the corresponding uncorrupted image. The same random points generated for symbolic reconstruction were employed in this process. To this end, these random points were first converted into a binary image. This image was smoothed by a Gaussian filter, and the intensity values were rescaled so that the maximum intensity value equals to the mean of the non-zero pixels in the corresponding uncorrupted image.

Examples of background subtracted projection images and corresponding centerline segmentations at varying levels of corruption were shown in Fig. 1.

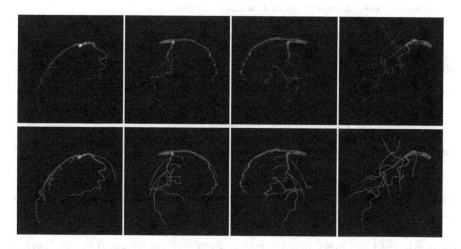

Fig. 1. Examples of the projection images at different corruption levels and from different views. (a)–(d) Projection images at 0%, 10%, 20%, and 30% corruption levels, respectively. (e)–(h) The centerline segmentations provided for the symbolic reconstruction were overlaid on the corresponding projection images.

Public Challenge Input Data. Finally, after generation of the projection domain data (i.e. images and centerline points) and artificial corruption thereof we provide the following data set as designated input to candidate reconstruction algorithms:

- **Background-subtracted projection images**: We provide background subtracted line-integral data of the contrasted coronary arteries at varying levels of corruption. The data is stored as meta-image [13] with detached headers. For analytic, FDK-type [14] reconstruction algorithms, we provide pre-processed versions of the line-integral images in the same format.
- **Densely sampled projection domain centerline points**: Projection domain centerlines at the four corruption levels are provided in separate text files, where the horizontal and vertical detector coordinates of a particular centerline point are whitespace separated and occupy one row each.
- **Cardiac phase data**: The relative cardiac phases are stored in a simple text file. The phases are periodic and in the interval $[0, 1]$, where $0 \equiv 1$ represents a phase at the end of ventricular diastole.
- **Projection matrices**: We provide projection matrices $\boldsymbol{P}_i \in \mathbb{R}^{3 \times 4}$ that encode the imaging geometry [15] and map from 3D world to 2D image coordinates. The matrix entries are stored as floats in a single binary file containing the 133 matrices in row-major order.

For a more detailed description of the provided data kindly refer to the particular section of this manuscript or the *CoronARe* challenge homepage[1], where we also link to exemplary code that provides guidance on how to handle the data.

2.3   Evaluation Protocol and Ranking

Tomographic Reconstruction. Scoring of tomographic reconstructions relies on *3D volumetric overlap*.

The input volume arising from tomographic reconstruction is repeatedly binarized using a sweeping threshold within the interval $[0, 255]$ [6]. The binary volume is then compared to the segmentation mask of the ground-truth morphology using the Dice similarity coefficient [16], a common two-sided measure for the overlap of two binary images ranging from zero (no overlap) to one (perfect match). As the final score, it selects the best value over all thresholds.

Symbolic Reconstruction. Scoring of symbolic centerline reconstructions relies on *3D reconstruction overlap curves*.

For a particular combination of ground truth and test centerline points, $\mathcal{P}_\mathcal{G}$ and $\mathcal{P}_\mathcal{S}$, respectively, the procedure is as follows.

To assess the overlap of a input reconstruction with the 3D ground truth we use a sweeping distance threshold $t_O \in [t_{\min}, t_{\max}]$ rather than the vessel

---

[1] Visit https://www5.cs.fau.de/research/software/coronare/.

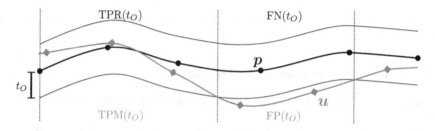

Fig. 2. Schematic illustration of the 3D reconstruction overlap curve computation. 3D points of the test and ground truth centerlines are labeled as true and false positives or negatives depending on the sweeping test distance t_O.

diameter. Given a distance t_O, every point of the ground truth $\boldsymbol{p} \in \mathcal{P_G}$ is marked as belonging to the set $\mathrm{TPR}(t_O)$ of true positives of the reference if there is at least one point $\boldsymbol{u} \in \mathcal{P_S}$ satisfying $d(\boldsymbol{p}, \boldsymbol{u}) < t_O$ and to the set $\mathrm{FN}(t_O)$ of false negatives otherwise. Points of the reconstruction $\boldsymbol{u}$ are labeled as belonging to the set $\mathrm{TPM}(t_O)$ of true positives of the tested method if there is at least one ground truth point $\boldsymbol{p}$ satisfying $d(\boldsymbol{u}, \boldsymbol{p}) < t_O$ and to the set $\mathrm{FP}(t_O)$ of false positives otherwise. An schematic of the labeling process is provided in Fig. 2. The overlap for a certain distance can then be computed as

$$O(t_O) = \frac{|\mathrm{TPM}(t_O)| + |\mathrm{TPR}(t_O)|}{|\mathrm{TPM}(t_O)| + |\mathrm{TPR}(t_O)| + |\mathrm{FN}(t_O)| + |\mathrm{FP}(t_O)|} \ . \tag{1}$$

Similar to the Dice score, the overlap measure ranges from zero (no overlap) to one (perfect match). With increasing distance thresholds the measure increases monotonically. A simple score that reflects the overall quality of a reconstruction is the area under the overlap curve

$$\tilde{O} = \frac{1}{t_{\max} - t_{\min}} \int_{t_{\min}}^{t_{\max}} O(t) \ \mathrm{d}t \tag{2}$$

that, again, ranges from zero to one indicating no to perfect overlap, respectively. A reasonable choice may be $(t_{\min}, t_{\max}) = (0 \, \mathrm{mm}, 1 \, \mathrm{mm})$.

2.4 Ranking

Our challenge design accommodates symbolic (i.e. centerline only) and tomographic coronary artery reconstruction. As the output of algorithms from both categories is substantially different, we perform a separate ranking of symbolic and tomographic algorithms.

Particularly, we select the best tomographic and symbolic methods with respect to overall reconstruction performance (averaged over all input data corruption levels) and with respect to clean data reconstruction performance.

Currently, there is no separate category for methods that incorporate external information, e.g. by using learning-based algorithms. The organizers emphasize that, in such cases, the XCAT anatomy must be excluded from the training and validation set.

2.5 Submission Guidelines and Formats

Partial participation (e.g. tomographic reconstruction, clean data only) is possible.

Although we provide full rotational angiography data, we highly encourage the participation of algorithms that do not operate on the complete data set, such as reconstruction from bi-plane data that is artificially created from the provided sequence.

The winners of the first phase of *CoronARe* were announced during an oral session at the *Reconstruction of Moving Body Organs (RAMBO)*[2] workshop that was held in conjunction with the *20*[th] *International Conference on Medical Image Computing and Computer Assisted Intervention (MICCAI) 2017*[3]. Evaluation within *CoronARe* is fully automated as it hosted using Kitware's Covalic [17]. Consequently, data download, result submission, and ranking remains possible even after the official completion of the first phase.

Submission formats for tomographic and symbolic reconstructions are held as simple as possible. For tomographic data we rely on the previously established *CAVAREV* format. For symbolic reconstruction we use a simple text file format where the coordinates of every 3D centerline point are whitespace separated and occupy one row each.

For a more detailed description of the submission file formats including example code for the tomographic format kindly refer to the *CoronARe* challenge homepage (see footnote 1).

3 Discussion and Outlook

We are aware and convinced of the fact that ranking of coronary artery reconstruction methods ultimately is most meaningful on clinical patient data, as such data imposes difficulties that are not sufficiently captured by in silico phantoms, such as anatomical variations (i.e. generalization). However, there is no joint benchmark for tomographic and symbolic reconstruction, even in a simple, controlled experimental setup. Moreover, the effects of corrupted projection domain data onto the reconstruction quality are not yet sufficiently understood. This challenge is meant to overcome these shortcomings, and to have a better understanding of the problem for future challenges that should be carried out on clinical data.

In conclusion, this challenge constitutes yet another effort in providing data and means of objective comparison. We hope to publish our findings of this first submission phase in a comprehensive journal article, ranking methods of

---

[2] Visit https://sites.google.com/view/miccai-rambo2017/home.

[3] Visit http://www.miccai2017.org/.

the current state-of-the-art. In tomographic reconstruction, we would be particularly interested in understanding how motion compensation strategies compare to algebraic methods that exploit prior knowledge on image appearance. When considering symbolic reconstruction methods, we believe that a comparison between bi-plane and multi-view reconstruction algorithms is of substantial interest.

Both data and submission will remain available even after closure of the initial submission phase. We hope this data to be helpful in future publications of peers, ideally, as a highly competitive benchmark of tomographic and symbolic coronary artery reconstruction algorithms.

Acknowledgement. The authors would like to thank Zach Mullen, Kitware, for his support in hosting this challenge.

References

1. Nichols, M., Townsend, N., Scarborough, P., Rayner, M.: Cardiovascular disease in Europe: epidemiological update. Eur. Heart J. **34**(39), 3028–3034 (2013)
2. Go, A.S., Mozaffarian, D., Roger, V.L., Benjamin, E.J., Berry, J.D., Blaha, M.J., Dai, S., Ford, E.S., Fox, C.S., Franco, S., et al.: Heart disease and stroke statistics - 2014 update. Circulation **129**(3) (2014)
3. Mark, D.B., Berman, D.S., Budoff, M.J., Carr, J.J., Gerber, T.C., Hecht, H.S., Hlatky, M.A., Hodgson, J.M., Lauer, M.S., Miller, J.M., et al.: ACCF/ACR/AHA/NASCI/SAIP/SCAI/SCCT 2010 expert consensus document on coronary computed tomographic angiography. Catheter Cardiovasc. Interv. **76**(2), E1–E42 (2010)
4. Gollapudi, R.R., Valencia, R., Lee, S.S., Wong, G.B., Teirstein, P.S., Price, M.J.: Utility of three-dimensional reconstruction of coronary angiography to guide percutaneous coronary intervention. Catheter Cardiovasc. Interv. **69**(4), 479–482 (2007)
5. Eng, M.H., Hudson, P.A., Klein, A.J., Chen, S.J., Kim, M.S., Groves, B.M., Messenger, J.C., Wink, O., Carroll, J.D., Garcia, J.A.: Impact of three dimensional in-room imaging (3DCA) in the facilitation of percutaneous coronary interventions. J. Cardiol. Vasc. Med. **1**(1), 1 (2013)
6. Rohkohl, C., Lauritsch, G., Keil, A., Hornegger, J.: CAVAREV-an open platform for evaluating 3D and 4D cardiac vasculature reconstruction. Phys. Med. Biol. **55**(10), 2905 (2010)
7. Çimen, S., Gooya, A., Grass, M., Frangi, A.F.: Reconstruction of coronary arteries from X-ray angiography: a review. Med. Image Anal. **32**, 46–68 (2016)
8. Dehkordi, M.T., Sadri, S., Doosthoseini, A.: A review of coronary vessel segmentation algorithms. J. Med. Sig. Sens. **1**(1), 49 (2011)
9. Unberath, M., Taubmann, O., Hell, M., Achenbach, S., Maier, A.: Symmetry, outliers, and geodesics in coronary artery centerline reconstruction from rotational angiography. Med. Phys. (2017, in press)
10. Segars, W.P., Sturgeon, G., Mendonca, S., Grimes, J., Tsui, B.M.W.: 4D XCAT phantom for multimodality imaging research. Med. Phys. **37**(9), 4902–4915 (2010)
11. Çimen, S., Gooya, A., Ravikumar, N., Taylor, Z.A., Frangi, A.F.: Reconstruction of coronary artery centrelines from X-ray angiography using a mixture of student's t-distributions. In: Ourselin, S., Joskowicz, L., Sabuncu, M.R., Unal, G., Wells, W. (eds.) MICCAI 2016. LNCS, vol. 9902, pp. 291–299. Springer, Cham (2016). doi:10.1007/978-3-319-46726-9_34

12. Unberath, M., Aichert, A., Achenbach, S., Maier, A.: Consistency-based respiratory motion estimation in rotational angiography. Med. Phys. (2017, in press)
13. Kitware: MetaIO Documentation (2014). https://itk.org/Wiki/ITK/MetaIO/Documentation. Accessed 9 June 2017
14. Feldkamp, L.A., Davis, L.C., Kress, J.W.: Practical cone-beam algorithm. J. Opt. Soc. Am. A **1**(6), 612–619 (1984)
15. Hartley, R., Zisserman, A.: Multiple View Geometry in Computer Vision, 2nd edn. Cambridge University Press, Cambridge (2004)
16. Sørensen, T.: A method of establishing groups of equal amplitude in plant sociology based on similarity of species and its application to analyses of the vegetation on danish commons. Biol. Skr. **5**, 1–34 (1948)
17. Kitware: Colvalic. https://challenge.kitware.com/. Accessed 9 July 2017

Freehand Ultrasound Image Simulation with Spatially-Conditioned Generative Adversarial Networks

Yipeng Hu[1,2(✉)], Eli Gibson[1], Li-Lin Lee[3], Weidi Xie[2], Dean C. Barratt[1], Tom Vercauteren[1], and J. Alison Noble[2]

[1] Centre for Medical Image Computing, University College London, London, UK
yipeng.hu@ucl.ac.uk
[2] Institute of Biomedical Engineering, University of Oxford, Oxford, UK
[3] Department of Diagnostic Imaging, Royal Free London NHS Foundation Trust, London, UK

Abstract. Sonography synthesis has a wide range of applications, including medical procedure simulation, clinical training and multimodality image registration. In this paper, we propose a machine learning approach to simulate ultrasound images at given 3D spatial locations (relative to the patient anatomy), based on conditional generative adversarial networks (GANs). In particular, we introduce a novel neural network architecture that can sample anatomically accurate images conditionally on spatial position of the (real or mock) freehand ultrasound probe. To ensure an effective and efficient spatial information assimilation, the proposed spatially-conditioned GANs take calibrated pixel coordinates in global physical space as conditioning input, and utilise residual network units and shortcuts of conditioning data in the GANs' discriminator and generator, respectively. Using optically tracked B-mode ultrasound images, acquired by an experienced sonographer on a fetus phantom, we demonstrate the feasibility of the proposed method by two sets of quantitative results: distances were calculated between corresponding anatomical landmarks identified in the held-out ultrasound images and the simulated data at the same locations unseen to the networks; a usability study was carried out to distinguish the simulated data from the real images. In summary, we present what we believe are state-of-the-art visually realistic ultrasound images, simulated by the proposed GAN architecture that is stable to train and capable of generating plausibly diverse image samples.

1 Introduction

Realistic simulation of medical ultrasound images is at the centre of many computer-assisted medical imaging innovations, such as simulating obstetric examination procedures to facilitate sonographer training [1] and simulating intra-operative images from pre-operative images to enable multimodality image data fusion for surgical planning and guidance [2]. However, one of the ultrasound-specific difficulties in modelling the imaging process is that significant variation during image acquisition comes from unquantified sources of uncertainty.

© Springer International Publishing AG 2017
M.J. Cardoso et al. (Eds.): CMMI/RAMBO/SWITCH 2017, LNCS 10555, pp. 105–115, 2017.
DOI: 10.1007/978-3-319-67564-0_11

Physics-based simulation methods for synthesising ultrasound images face significant challenges. Solving large-scale partial differential equations for modelling the nonlinear wave propagation requires substantial computational resource, often infeasible for interactive use. For instance, state-of-the-art simulation needs to make many simplifying assumptions such as ray tracing, static scattering map and requires *a prior* segmentation in order to obtain real-time simulations, e.g. [3]. Furthermore, it is particularly challenging to simulate ultrasound images for individual subjects as acoustic properties of patient-specific soft tissue are in general infeasible to obtain. *In vivo* soft tissue properties are deformable, heterogeneous, and may contain pathologies of interest, all of which vary significantly in individual patients. To the best of our knowledge, there has little published modelling technique available to model acoustic patterns in sonography due to variation at cellular level while modelling motion and deformation at organ level remains on-going research [3].

Manikin based simulators highly depend on the quality of the materials (e.g. realistic acoustic and viscoelastic properties) and the pre-designed fixed anatomy, and hence remains an expensive option. Real patient image databases have also been used in commercial ultrasound simulators. Building these databases relies on nontrivial effort in collecting comprehensive patient cohort, clinical problems and usage cases. There is little published detailed methodology or available data library for research validation. Both methods are therefore limited to pre-defined clinical scenarios for training purposes and are not directly applicable for patient-specific applications such as registering to the pre-operative images of the same patient.

Alternatively, machine learning methods potentially can overcome these restrictions by inferring from real image data. In this work, we are primarily interested in obstetric examination, where freehand ultrasound simulators are increasingly used for training sonographers [1]. Ideal for this clinical scenario, images of the fetus need to be simulated (inferred) at new spatial locations relative to patient anatomy. We argue that fully supervised approaches, such as regression, for predicting ultrasound images are problematic because acquisition-position-independent uncertainties in acquiring training data are both inevitable and significant, such as those caused by the distribution of the acoustic coupling agent, patient motion and other user-dependent variation. For instances, acoustic shadows and refraction artefacts could occur at various regions within the ultrasound fields of view acquired at the same physical location; the speckle pattern changes due to the flow of fluid (e.g. blood) in living tissue. As a result, regression models often lead to blurred averages of nearby training data (see an example in Fig. 5) and instantiations that contain sonographic characteristics cannot be easily sampled. Therefore, we propose to use generative adversarial networks (GANs) [4, 5] to model the image distribution as opposed to predicting one single "best" image. From the trained neural network, instances can then be sampled to retain realistic features learned from training data. Furthermore, neural-network-based models can readily generate simulated images on-the-fly without extra engineering effort or specialised hardware.

Using ultrasound image and optical tracking data acquired on a fetus phantom, we summarise our contribution in this proof-of-concept study as follows: (a) proposing a novel and stable network architecture for generative modelling of ultrasound images; (b) demonstrating the feasibility of conditional GANs to simulate fetal ultrasound images at locations unseen to the networks; (c) quantifying the proposed method using clinically relevant anatomical regions and landmarks; (d) producing state-of-the-art visually realistic ultrasound simulation results verified by a usability study.

2 Method

2.1 Spatially-Conditioned Generative Adversarial Learning

In this work, we propose to model the conditional distribution $P_{im}(\mathbf{x}|\mathbf{y})$ of the ultrasound images $\mathbf{x} \sim P_{im}(\mathbf{x}|\mathbf{y})$, given spatial locations $\mathbf{y} \sim P_{loc}(\mathbf{y})$ with respect to a fixed physical reference obtained from a position tracking device. The experiment and data acquisition details are provided in Sect. 2.3. The ultrasound simulator can then be constructed by optimising the latent parameters θ_G of a *generator* neural network $G(\mathbf{z}, \mathbf{y})$, so it maps independent unit Gaussian noise $\mathbf{z} \sim N(\mathbf{z})$ to the observed image space for each given spatial location $\mathbf{y}$.

In a zero-sum minimax optimisation framework described in GANs [4], the generator is optimised through the *discriminator* neural network $D(\mathbf{x}, \mathbf{y})$ with latent parameters θ_D, which outputs a scalar likelihood classifying the input as true or false, i.e. real or fake ultrasound image at location $\mathbf{y}$. This is achieved by jointly optimising the cost functions of the discriminator and the generator, $J^{(D)}$ and $J^{(G)}$, respectively:

$$J^{(D)} = -\frac{1}{2}\mathbb{E}_{(\mathbf{x},\mathbf{y})\sim P_{data}} \log D(\mathbf{x}, \mathbf{y}) - \frac{1}{2}\mathbb{E}_{\mathbf{z}\sim N, \mathbf{y}\sim P_{loc}} \log\left(1 - D(G(\mathbf{z}, \mathbf{y}), \mathbf{y})\right) \tag{1}$$

and

$$J^{(G)} = -\frac{1}{2}\mathbb{E}_{\mathbf{z}\sim N, \mathbf{y}\sim P_{loc}} \log D(G(\mathbf{z}, \mathbf{y}), \mathbf{y}) \tag{2}$$

where $\mathbb{E}$ is the statistical expectation. Using sample pairs from data distribution $(\mathbf{x}, \mathbf{y}) \sim P_{data}(\mathbf{x}, \mathbf{y})$, parameters θ_D and θ_G are each updated once in every iteration to decrease the values of respective $J^{(D)}$ and $J^{(G)}$ cost functions. Conceptually, optimising $J^{(G)}$ aims to enable $G(\mathbf{z}, \mathbf{y})$ to generate samples that the discriminator classifies as true images; while $J^{(D)}$ is optimised, in an adversarial manner, to "correctly" classify the generator produced images $G(\mathbf{z}, \mathbf{y})$ and samples from the training data set $\mathbf{x}$ as false and true images, respectively. Once convergence is reached, the generator is expected to generate samples from a distribution approximating the conditional data distribution, by only sampling from the $N(\mathbf{z})$ with a given spatial location. The implementation details of the two networks are given in the following sections.

2.2 Network Architecture

Central to our proposed method is to assimilate the spatial information in an effective and balanced manner, so the non-stationary minimax optimisation can produce images conditioned on the given spatial locations while variations, captured by the input noise, are still preserved. Although, in theory, the physical transformation directly obtained from the tracking could be added to the inputs of the generator and the discriminator for conditioning purpose [4], we found in practice simple concatenation of the transformation vectors in terms of rotation and translation was not effective. The neural networks failed to converge to generating images containing spatially correct anatomy at the given locations. Therefore, we propose: (1) to use calibrated 3D physical coordinates of the image pixels as the input conditioning data (Fig. 1 Left); (2) to concatenate the resized x-, y- and z coordinate grids (as three channels) before each up-sampling layer in the generator; (3) to adopt residual network units [6] throughout the discriminator with the conditioning coordinates only being concatenated with input image. An overview of the network architecture is sketched in Fig. 1.

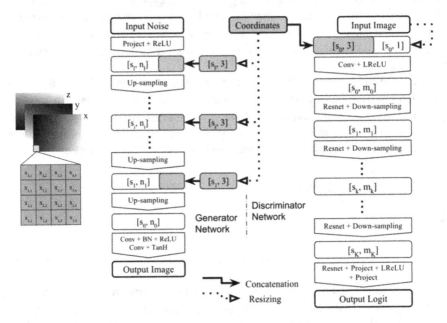

Fig. 1. Left: an illustration of the calibrated physical x-, y- and z coordinates of image pixels, contained in three channels; Right: an overview of the neural network architecture used in the proposed conditional generative adversarial networks, where s_i and s_k are sizes of the feature maps while n_i and m_k are numbers of channels. See details in Sect. 2.2.

In the generator network, 100 random Gaussian noise with zero mean and unit variance is first projected with rectified linear units (ReLU) to feature maps having a small size s_1 and n_1 initial channels. Then the "up-sampling" layers double the size of the previous feature maps and halve the number of channels, until the size of the image is reached. Each $i^{th}(i = 1, \ldots, I)$ up-sampling layer consists of a transposed convolution with a 2×2 stride and a convolution (conv), both with batch normalisation (BN) and ReLU. The last layer has a convolution with BN and ReLU, and a second convolution with hyperbolic tangent function (TanH) as activation without BN to retain true data statistics and range [5]. The three conditioning channels containing x-, y- and z pixel coordinates are resized to the respective sizes and concatenated to the feature maps just before each up-sampling (the image-sized coordinate channels were therefore not used directly in the generator). All the convolutional layers in the generator have a 3×3 kernel size.

The discriminator network accepts a concatenation of an input image and its corresponding three-channel pixel coordinates, mapping to feature maps of the same size and m_0 initial channels by a convolution with leaky ReLU (LReLU) as activation function, suggested in [5]. Pairs of residual network unit (Resnet) and "down-sampling" layer halve the size of the previous feature maps and double the number of channels. Each $k^{th}(k = 1, \ldots, K)$ Resnet layer has two convolutions both with BN and LReLU, and an identity mapping for shortcut. Each down-sampling layer has a 2×2 stride convolution with BN and LReLU. The final Logit with one-sided label smoothing [7] is outputted after an additional Resnet, two projections (to a single image size and to a scalar, respectively) with a nonlinear LReLU in between. All the convolutional layers in the discriminator also have a 3×3 kernel size, with an exception of the first one having a larger 5×5 kernel.

2.3 Validation Experiment

An approximately one hour scan of an anatomically realistic fetus ultrasound examination phantom ("SPACE FAN-ST", Kyoto Kagaku Co., Ltd, Kyoto, Japan) was performed by a Reporting Sonographer with more than ten years' experience. As illustrated in Fig. 2, the abdominal probe (Ultrasonix 4DC7-3/40, BK Ultrasound, BC, Canada) was tracked by an optical tracker (Polaris Spectra, NDI Europe, Radolfzell, Germany). The ultrasound images and tracking data were timestamped by NifTK (niftk.org) [8]. The data were acquired in four sessions at neurological, cardiological, abdominal and fetal profile regions, following standard NHS Fetal Anomaly Screening Programme.

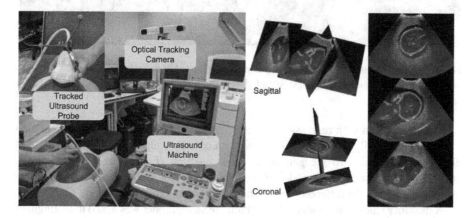

Fig. 2. Left: the laboratory setup for acquiring the ultrasound image and optical tracking data; Right: example ultrasound frames plotted both in 3d (using calibrated tracking data) and in 2d.

A total of 26,396 image frames were normalised to an intensity range of $[-1, 1]$ and were down-sampled to 160×120 pixels in this study, only images containing anatomical structures being used in this study for computational consideration. The physical pixel coordinates were calibrated based on a pinhead-based calibration method [9], before being normalised to zero-mean and unit variance. The calibration procedure acquired 87 tracked 2D ultrasound images of a fixed pinhead at different angles and positions to estimate the relative transformation from local image coordinates to global physical coordinates together with the in-plane resolution.

The proposed GANs-based ultrasound simulator was implemented with Tensor-Flow™ and trained on a 12 GB NVIDIA® Tesla™ K40 GPU, using the Adam optimiser with learning rate set to 0.0002, first- and second moment estimates set to 0.5 and 0.999, respectively. The results presented in this paper was obtained with a minibatch size of 36, no weight decay or clipping, $I = 4$ down-sampling- and $K = 5$ up-sampling layers, 512 and 32 initial channels for the generator and the discriminator, respectively.

To assess the anatomical fidelity of the simulation, clinically interesting landmarks, including crux of four heart chambers, centre of stomach, cord insertion, mid-line echo, cavum septum pellucidum and nasal tip on profile, were identified in both the held-out real images and the simulated images generated from a 10-fold cross-validation experiment (see examples in Fig. 3). Images were also excluded from training data if the tracked transformation (in rotation and translation) is within 95% confidence interval [10] of any transformation in those of held-out test data.

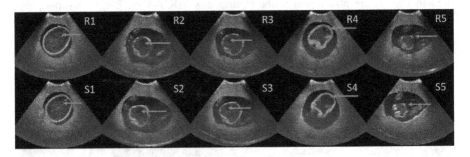

Fig. 3. Example anatomical landmarks (orange arrows) used in this work, between real images (top row, R1-5) and simulated images sampled at the same locations (bottom row, S1-5). (Color figure online)

For comparison with regression-like approaches, two additional models were also trained: (1) a heavily-supervised GANs with an equally-weighted L^2-norm regularisation term [11] added to the generator's cost function (Eq. 2), with other settings unchanged; (2) a regression model of the same generator architecture, directly minimising L^2-norm of the difference between generated- and training images.

A usability study was conducted, in which the sonographer was asked to distinguish whether the images are simulated or real. Randomly sampled 100 generated simulations together with 100 real ultrasound images were shuffled, before being displayed full-screen on a 15-inch monitor. To further quantify the GANs' ability to generate realistic content at different spatial frequencies, the experiment was repeated while a Gaussian filter was applied with different kernel sizes (standard deviation σ ranged from 2 to 0 mm, with zero indicating that the original images produced by the network and the original real images were used directly).

3   Results

The generator network can produce more than 1 k frames per second (fps) on the same GPU and ~60 fps on an Intel® Core™ i7 CPU, well satisfying real-time requirement. The examples of simulated ultrasound images at locations unseen to the networks are provided in Fig. 4, together with corresponding ground-truth images at the same spatial locations. Verified by the same sonographer who acquired the data, 120 landmarks were identified in the held-out real images. Among the randomly sampled 120 simulated images, 3 (2.5%) were considered as producing incorrect or unrecognisable regions, while 47 (39.2%) simulated images contain recognisable anatomical regions but no clearly identifiable corresponding landmarks. From the remaining 70 (58.3%) image pairs, 2D distances were calculated between the corresponding landmarks from simulated- and ground-truth images, yielding a mean 6.1 ± 1.2 mm error.

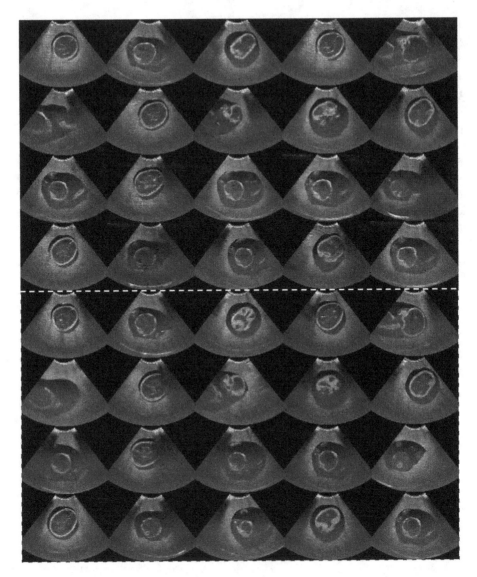

Fig. 4. Top four rows: examples of randomly-sampled ultrasound image simulations at unseen spatial locations; bottom four rows: real ultrasound images at the same locations in the validation data set.

Figure 5 contains example simulated images from (1) the GANs trained with heavily supervised regularisation and (2) the regression model, both described in Sect. 2.3. It demonstrates that, compared with the images from the proposed simulator, the apparent blurring effect is predominant from the two more supervised learning approaches with inferior visual features and details.

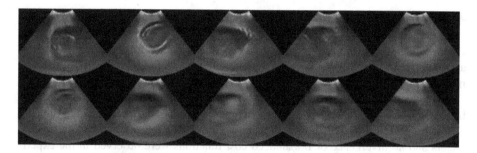

Fig. 5. Examples of simulations using the supervised cost functions: (1) Top row: the images sampled from the trained GANs with heavily supervised regularisation; (2) Bottom row: the regression predicted images with the L^2-norm objective function (see details in Sect. 2.3).

We report an interesting result from the usability study described in Sect. 2.3. The sonographer was able to correctly distinguish 124 (62%) and 162 (81%) test images, with Gaussian filtering ($\sigma = 1$ mm) and without filtering ($\sigma = 0$ mm), respectively. The difference may partly be explained by the network-related high frequency artefacts (e.g. checkboard artefacts in transposed convolution [12]) being filtered with larger kernels. We note that any Gaussian kernel with a size larger than $\sigma = 1.5$ mm was deemed too blur to avoid random guess (approaching 50% correction rate).

To further investigate the variance learned by the generative models, Fig. 6 illustrates the simulated images by only sampling the prior noise $\mathbf{z}$ with fixed conditioning $\mathbf{y}$. It shows that, also found in Fig. 4, changes in detailed intensity patterns, positions of shadows and artefacts, and minor anatomical variation may be captured by modelling the conditional distribution of ultrasound images.

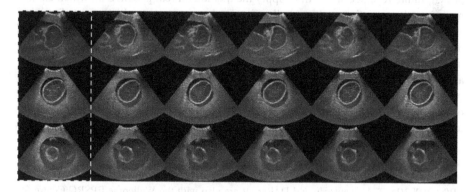

Fig. 6. Examples of randomly-sampled ultrasound image simulations at the same spatial locations (rows) with the first column displaying the ground-truth real ultrasound images acquired at the same locations.

4 Conclusion and Discussion

Based on both the qualitative and quantitative results reported in this paper, we present a promising approach for generative representation learning of freehand ultrasound images in fetal examination.

Our experience suggests that the proposed GAN architecture, together with the calibrated physical coordinates as conditioning input, not only reduces the training time but also stabilises the convergence, e.g. the training was relatively insensitive to hyperparameters and no divergence or imbalanced cost functions were observed in the experiments. This is probably a result of the presumably simplified training objective and better supervision from the conditioning information at different resolution levels. However, further results are needed to draw a comprehensive conclusion.

There has been evidence of *mode-collapse* at some physical locations. Arguably, it may not be critical in this application that aims to produce high quality samples instead of complete coverage of the image distribution. A full investigation of this well-recognised problem is beyond the scope of the current work, and remains an open research question, e.g. [7]. Minor *underfitting* has been observed with the presented GANs, evidenced by the fact that the samples drawn from locations in the training set are very similar (both in subjective appearance and quantitative landmark distance) to those found in testing. Therefore, we believe that, considering the variation in the learned conditional distribution, the reported landmark error reflects the modelling ability of generating spatially coherent anatomical features, rather than an indication of copying nearest training data.

Although deformation was commonplace during the experiment due to probe pressure and the soft mattress of the surgical bed on which the deformable phantom was placed, future research will aim to apply the method on real patient data which exhibit more complex variation such as challenging fetal movement. A wider range of training and test data (e.g. acquired by non-experts) may need to be included for the purpose of training less experienced users, and investigating other types of conditioning information (e.g. ultrasound parameters and temporal variation) could also improve the interactive capacity of the proposed simulator. We would also like to note that, although an optical tracker was used in this validation, the trained simulator may be feasible to run on consumer-grade mobile devices equipped with inexpensive inertial measurement units.

Acknowledgement. This work was supported by the Wellcome Trust, CRUK and the EPSRC (EP/M020533/1; C28070/A19985; WT101957; 203145Z/16/Z; NS/A000027/1; EP/M020533/1; EP/N026993/1). T. Vercauteren and D. Barratt are also with the Wellcome/EPSRC Centre for Interventional and Surgical Sciences. The authors would like to thank Dr Matt Clarkson, Dr Steve Thompson, and Dr Francisco Vasconcelos from UCL for assistance with data collection. The source code used in this work is available on NiftyNet platform (niftynet.io) under an Apache 2.0 license.

References

1. Maul, H., et al.: Ultrasound simulators: experience with the SonoTrainer and comparative review of other training systems. Ultrasound Obstet. Gynecol. **24**(5), 581–585 (2004)
2. Wein, W., Khamene, A., Clevert, D.-A., Kutter, O., Navab, N.: Simulation and fully automatic multimodal registration of medical ultrasound. In: Ayache, N., Ourselin, S., Maeder, A. (eds.) MICCAI 2007. LNCS, vol. 4791, pp. 136–143. Springer, Heidelberg (2007). doi: 10.1007/978-3-540-75757-3_17
3. Burger, B., et al.: Real-time GPU-based ultrasound simulation using deformable mesh models. IEEE Trans. Med. Imaging **32**(3), 609–618 (2013)
4. Goodfellow, I., et al.: Generative adversarial nets. In: Advances in Neural Information Processing Systems, pp. 2672–2680 (2014)
5. Radford, A., Metz, L., Chintala, S.: Unsupervised representation learning with deep convolutional generative adversarial networks. arXiv preprint arXiv:1511.06434 (2015)
6. He, K., et al.: Deep residual learning for image recognition. In: Proceedings of the IEEE Conference on Computer Vision and Pattern Recognition, pp. 770–778 (2016)
7. Salimans, T., et al.: Improved techniques for training GANs. In: Advances in Neural Information Processing Systems, pp. 2234–2242 (2016)
8. Clarkson, M.J., et al.: The NifTK software platform for image-guided interventions: platform overview and NiftyLink messaging. Int. J. Comput. Assist. Radiol. Surg. **10**(3), 301–316 (2015)
9. Hu, Y., et al.: Development and phantom validation of a 3-D-ultrasound-guided system for targeting MRI-visible lesions during transrectal prostate biopsy. IEEE Trans. Bio-med. Eng. **64**(4), 946 (2017)
10. Elfring, R., de la Fuente, M., Radermacher, K.: Assessment of optical localizer accuracy for computer aided surgery systems. Comput. Aided Surg. **15**(1–3), 1–12 (2010)
11. Pathak, D., et al.: Context encoders: feature learning by inpainting. In: Proceedings of the IEEE Conference on Computer Vision and Pattern Recognition, pp. 2536–2544 (2016)
12. Odena, A., Dumoulin, V., Olah, C.: Deconvolution and checkerboard artifacts. Distill **1**(10), e3 (2016)

Context-Sensitive Super-Resolution for Fast Fetal Magnetic Resonance Imaging

Steven McDonagh[1(✉)], Benjamin Hou[1], Amir Alansary[1], Ozan Oktay[1], Konstantinos Kamnitsas[1], Mary Rutherford[2], Jo V. Hajnal[2], and Bernhard Kainz[1,2]

[1] Biomedical Image Analysis Group, Imperial College London, London, UK
steven.mcdonagh@imperial.ac.uk
[2] Division of Imaging Sciences and Biomedical Engineering,
Kings College London, London, UK

Abstract. 3D Magnetic Resonance Imaging (MRI) is often a trade-off between fast but low-resolution image acquisition and highly detailed but slow image acquisition. Fast imaging is required for targets that move to avoid motion artefacts. This is in particular difficult for fetal MRI. Spatially independent upsampling techniques, which are the state-of-the-art to address this problem, are error prone and disregard contextual information. In this paper we propose a context-sensitive upsampling method based on a residual convolutional neural network model that learns organ specific appearance and adopts semantically to input data allowing for the generation of high resolution images with sharp edges and fine scale detail. By making contextual decisions about appearance and shape, present in different parts of an image, we gain a maximum of structural detail at a similar contrast as provided by high-resolution data. We experiment on 145 fetal scans and show that our approach yields an increased PSNR of 1.25 dB when applied to under-sampled fetal data *cf.* baseline upsampling. Furthermore, our method yields an increased PSNR of 1.73 dB when utilizing under-sampled fetal data to perform brain volume reconstruction on motion corrupted captured data.

1 Introduction

Currently, 3D imaging of moving objects is limited by the time it takes to acquire a single image. The slower an imaging modality is, the more likely motion induced artefacts will occur within and between individual slices of a 3D volume. Very fast imaging modalities like Computed Tomography are not always applicable because of harmful ionising radiation, and ultrasound often suffers from poor image quality. Thus, Magnetic Resonance Imaging (MRI) is usually the modality of choice when; large fields of view, high anatomical detail, and non-invasive imaging is required. MRI is often applied to image involuntary moving objects such as the beating heart and examination of the fetus in-utero. Motion compensation for cardiac imagining can be achieved through ECG gating. However, fetal targets do not provide options for gated or tracked image acquisition to compensate for motion. Thus motion compensation is performed during

© Springer International Publishing AG 2017
M.J. Cardoso et al. (Eds.): CMMI/RAMBO/SWITCH 2017, LNCS 10555, pp. 116–126, 2017.
DOI: 10.1007/978-3-319-67564-0_12

post-processing of oversampled input spaces, usually involving the acquisition of orthogonally oriented stacks of slices [8]. Oversampling with high resolution (HR) slices causes long scan times, which is uncomfortable and risky for patients like pregnant women. This limits the possible number of scan sequences during examination. However, improving image resolution is key to improving accuracy, understanding of anatomy and assessment of organ size and morphology. Imaging at lower resolution increases acquisition speed, thus partly mitigating the likelihood for motion between individual slices but at the cost of missing structural detail that could render the scan inappropriate for diagnostic purposes. Due to signal-to-noise ratio (SNR) limitations, the acquired slices are usually also *thick* compared to the in-plane resolution and thus negatively influence the visualization of anatomy in 3D.

Naïve up-sampling of fast but low resolution (LR) images is undesirable for the clinical practice, since results lack information. Information content cannot be increased by simply increasing the number of pixels with linear interpolation methods. Therefore, optimization-based super-resolution (SR) methods have been explored to generate rich volumetric information from oversampled input spaces. However, these methods are highly dependent on the quality and amount of input samples and depend on the choice of the objective function. Recent work, *e.g.* [4], on example-based SR has focused on incorporating additional prior image knowledge, and, in particular, deep neural networks have been employed to solve the single-image SR (SISR) problem. However, the majority of recent contributions typically place strong emphasis on natural images and therefore lack domain specific high-frequency detail prior knowledge [1].

Contribution: We present a novel approach to SISR in the context of motion compensation when using fast to acquire, low resolution volumes. Taking inspiration from recent investigation of network based SR for MRI modalities [15], we propose a network architecture with convolutional and transposed-convolutional layers and hypothesize that such a deep network architecture can be tailored to context sensitive applications, such as motion compensation of the fetal brain, and yield volume reconstruction improvements from low resolution input. Our network learns subject specific details from potentially motion corrupted input data and accurately reintroduces the expected fidelity allowing motion compensation and high quality reconstruction from fast low resolution input.

Our model is in particular data-adaptive since the upsampling is performed by learnable transposed-convolution layers instead of a fixed kernel. By performing the upsampling in the final layers of the network we avoid early redundant computation in a HR space, enabling a computational saving. Additionally by considering entire LR in-plane slice samples at training time, in comparison to image *patches*, we gain a large receptive field to enable the learning of spatial context, organ structure and anatomy.

We evaluate our method on 145 healthy fetal scans. The proposed approach shows improved qualitative results when compared visually to linear methods. Quantitative reconstruction performance, peak signal-to-noise-ratio (PSNR) and structural similarity index measure (SSIM) improve, accordingly. In particular, we reach comparable reconstruction quality with half as many data samples, thus half of the currently required scan time, when compared to motion compensated reconstruction from high-resolution image acquisition.

Related work: The topic of SR has received much attention in the literature and a large body of work exists however, historically, algorithms exhibiting good performance in 2D domains such as satellite or facial imagery, are not necessarily ideal for 3D medical imaging. This is partly due to domain specific effects such as loss of spatial information caused by motion during slow target acquisition. Various algorithms have been shown to produce leading results [14] in differing domains.

SISR accounts for missing image information by using previously observed examples to optimise the LR-HR mapping between images or patches. In the medical imaging domain, data-adaptive patch-based approaches to SISR reconstruction [7,13] have been shown to prevent the occurrence of well-known blurring effects, often found when using classical interpolation approaches. Interpolation techniques tend to increase the smoothness of images in an isotropic manner, however data-adaptive non-local methods allow for highly anisotropic reconstruction where required. In patch-based methods, the radius of 3D patch used to compute the similarity among voxels is often a free parameter and the choice of receptive field size typically affects computational cost when using iterative optimisation.

Learning based approaches also allow data-adaptive reconstruction and CNNs in particular have recently been successfully applied to context sensitive SISR for cardiac imaging. The work of [15] use a regression architecture based on [4] with a modified l_1 objective function. The approach performed SR in the slice-select direction of lowest MRI resolution, *i.e.*, one-dimensionally and utilized transposed convolutional layers at the start of the network architecture to perform the upsampling, *prior* to convolutions, thus learning high level features in latter layers on (spatially) large feature maps.

Two-dimensional SR is a popular research area in natural image processing due to many applications requiring enhancement of a visual experience while limiting the amount of raw data that needs to be recorded, transferred or stored. Recent network-based approaches such as SRGAN [12] apply Generative Adversarial Networks (GAN) to achieve large up-sampling factors of up to four.

Motion compensation for MRI volume reconstruction typically incorporates a SR component. However to the best of our knowledge state-of-the-art network based SR techniques, capable of learning problem and sensor specifics from available data have not been harnessed for the upsampling step found in Slice-to-Volume frameworks for the reconstruction task. In this work we investigate the accuracy advantages that such an approach can contribute to the example of fetal MRI volume reconstruction.

Contemporary SR components in MRI Slice-to-Volume reconstruction (SVR) tasks perform optimisation based incremental updates to the HR volume estimate. To achieve this, the SR problem for volume reconstruction has been modelled directly by considering minimisation of an error norm function and use of Huber function statistics [5] or gradient-weighted averaging [10]. The ill-posed nature of modelling upsampling requires that the objective be regularised. Gholipour *et al.* [5] add a Tikhonov term to the cost for this purpose while Rousseau *et al.* [16–18] select a regularisation term that includes an approximation of Total Variation (TV) to better preserve edges. Tourbier *et al.* [21] apply fast convex optimization techniques for the SR problem also using an edge-preserving TV regularization. Murgasova *et al.* [11] used intensity matching and complete outlier removal for reconstruction. SR volume intensities are iteratively updated using the error gradients resulting from differences between simulated and observed slice samples. Transforming observed slice information to the upsampled volume space requires accurate yet potentially computationally expensive estimation of the sensor point spread function (PSF) and [8] developed a fast multi-GPU accelerated implementation for the task.

2   Method

The proposed approach implements a fully three-dimensional CNN architecture to infer upsampled MRI imagery, enabling HR input to be provided for subsequent SVR and motion compensation tasks. We define an architecture utilising 3D volumetric convolutions that have recently been shown to add value for medical imaging tasks considering 3D imagery [2,9]. Figure 1 provides a schematic of our upsampling network and architecture design details are provide in the **3D MRI CNN** subsection below. Figure 2 provides a schematic diagram indicating where the upsampling network component is implemented in a SVR reconstruction framework.

The architecture differs from recent network based MRI SR models [15] by generating feature maps in the LR image space *cf.* early redundant feature channel upsampling or fixed kernels [3], reducing memory and computation requirements while retaining the flexibility of learnable upsampling layers. As previously reported [19], early upsampling tends to introduce redundant computation in the

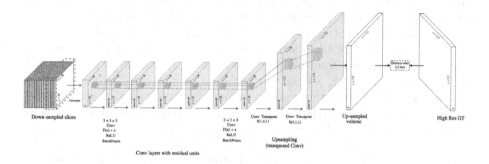

Fig. 1. Our proposed CNN network architecture for MRI super-resolution. See text for architecture details.

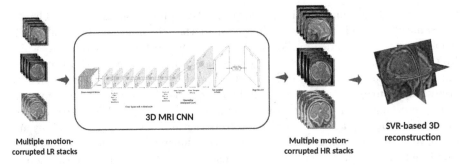

Fig. 2. The proposed framework for providing upsampled, high resolution input for motion correction and volume reconstruction.

HR space since no additional information is added into the model by performing transposed convolutions at an early stage of the architecture.

Our approach mitigates the acquisition quality cost of low resolution imagery by considering the problem of estimating a high dimensional $\mathbf{y} \in \mathbb{R}^M$, for a given observation $\mathbf{x} = f(y) \in \mathbb{R}^N$ where $(N \ll M)$. SR is an underdetermined inverse problem, and as such the function f performs a downsampling and is typically non-invertible. The low-dimensional observation $\mathbf{x}$ is mapped to the high-dimensional $\mathbf{y}$ by recovery through the MR image acquisition model [6], a series of operators such that: $\mathbf{x} = DBSM\mathbf{y} + \eta$ where M defines a spatial displacement, $e.g.$ due to motion, S is the slice selection operator, B is the point-spread function (PSF) used to blur the selected slice, D is a decimation operator, and η is a Rician noise model. We approximate solutions to this inverse problem by estimating $\phi(\mathbf{x}, \Theta)$ from the LR input such that a cost, defined between $\phi(\mathbf{x}, \Theta)$ and $\mathbf{y}$, is minimized. We estimate the parameters Θ using a CNN architecture with parameters Θ that parametrise network layers to model the distribution $p(y|x)$. Training samples are defined as $(\mathbf{x}_i, \mathbf{y}_i)$.

3D MRI CNN: In-plane, low-resolution MRI stacks are synthetically generated simply by filtering HR images with a Cosine Windowed Sinc blurring kernel followed by a decimation operator to provide LR-HR training pairs as input. Training samples consist of entire LR in-plane imagery with a volume defined by $z >= 1$ out-of-plane slices forming 3D volume training samples, providing contextual information from multiple slices. Here we report on experimental upsampling factors of ×2, ×4 and $z = 5$.

Our 3D-CNN architecture contains nine layers consisting of six convolutional layers, utilising standard ReLU activations and residual units, followed by two transposed-convolutional layers (with corresponding strides of two or four) and a final single-channel layer to build the full resolution output. The ReLU activation function has exhibited strong performance when upscaling both natural images [4] and MRI 3D volume data [15]. Intermediate feature maps $h_j^{(n)}$ at layer n are computed through convolutional kernels w_{kj}^n as $max(0, \Sigma_{k=1}^K h_k^{(n-1)} * w_{kj}^n) = h_j^n$ where $*$ is the convolutional operator. We follow the common frugal strategy [20] of applying small ($3 \times 3 \times 3$) convolution kernels and spending compute-budget alternatively on layer count to increase receptive field size.

By introducing two transposed convolution layers we perform the upscaling on in-plane sampling dimensions. In this manner, upscaling weights are learned specifically for the SR task where $(x \uparrow U_x) * w_j = h_j^0$ and $(h_1 \uparrow U_y) * w_j = h_j^1$ where $\uparrow$ is a zero-padding upscaling operator and $\{U_x, U_y\} = M/N$ are the in-plane upscaling factors. This allows for explicit optimization of the upsampling filters and facilitates training in an end-to-end manner for the SR task. By implementing trainable upsampling layers we improve upon the alternative strategy of initial independent linear upsampling, followed only by convolutional layers, as we gain an ability to learn upsampling weights specific to the SR task. In practice this often improves MRI image signal quality in image regions close to boundaries [15]. Residuals learned by the convolution layers and the upscaled transposed-convolutional output are used to reconstruct the final HR image. This allows the regression function to learn non-linearities such as the high frequency components of the signal.

Training involves evaluating the error function $\Psi_{l_2}(\cdot)$ that calculates the difference between the reconstructed HR images and the ground truth volumes that were down-sampled to provide training data. Model weights are updated using standard back-propagation and adaptive moment estimation. In comparison to modified l_1 losses [15] or recent *perceptual-quality* SR objective functions [12], we implement a standard voxel-wise l_2 loss function to provide gradient information and emphasize voxel-wise difference to the ground-truth. An implementation of our model training strategy is made available online[1].

Fetal Brain Volume Reconstruction: We combine our SR network with Slice-to-Volume registration (SVR) [8]. SVR requires multiple orthogonal stacks of 2D slices to provide improved reconstruction quality. By upsampling stacks prior to reconstruction we provide a means to acquire larger sets of low-resolution input. The motion-free 3D image is then reconstructed from the upsampled slices and motion-corrupted and misaligned areas are excluded during the reconstruction using an EM-based outliers rejection model.

3 Experiments

Data: We test our approach on clinical MR scans with varying gestational age. All scans have been ethically approved. The dataset contains 145 MR scans of healthy fetuses at gestational age between 20–25 weeks. The data has been acquired on a Philips Achieva 1.5T, the mother lying 20° tilt on the left side to avoid pressure on the inferior vena cava. Single-shot fast spin (ssFSE) T2-weighted sequences are used to acquire stacks of images that are aligned to the main axes of the fetus. Three to six stacks with a voxel size of

---

[1] https://github.com/DLTK.

1.25 mm × 1.25 mm × 2.5 mm per stack are acquired for the whole womb. Imagery is manually masked and cropped to isolate fetal brain regions.

Experimental details: We employ our 3D MRI network and separately two baseline SR strategies to upsample image stack inputs that serve as input to the SVR pipeline. SVR then performs motion compensation and volume reconstruction. We assess upsampled image quality directly and, additionally, investigate the effect of the proposed upsampling strategy on reconstruction quality, from the (initially) low resolution fetal data. We report three quantitative metrics: PSNR, structural similarity index (SSIM) and cross-correlation. In the first experiment, the data is randomly split into two subsets and used to train (100) and test (45) with our SR network. MRI stacks represent 46 individual patients and all image stacks, belonging to a particular patient, are found uniquely in either the train or test set. Images are cropped, intensity normalised and linearly downsampled by factors of 2 and 4 with respect to the in-plane stack axes. This resampling provides LR images to our network resulting in multiple training samples per volume with corresponding ground-truth label (HR source image). The network uses these training pairs to learn the LR to HR mapping. Note that image volume size choices introduce a trade-off between available contextual information and pragmatic memory constraints.

4   Evaluation and Results

Image Quality Assessments: We compare HR ground-truth 3D volumes with upsampled LR raw data by measuring PSNR, SSIM and cross-correlation. We report SSIM, in particular, due to the well-understood metric properties that afford assessment of local structure correlation and reduced noise sensitivity. LR test imagery is upsampled in-plane (X, Y) by factors of 2, 4 to align with target ground-truth resolution. Quality metrics in Fig. 3 report improvements observed for an image upsampling factor of 2. This provides initial evidence in support of our hypothesis; *learning problem and sensor specific deconvolutional filters to perform MRI stack upsampling is of benefit for subsequent resolution-sensitive tasks such as motion compensation and HR volume reconstruction.*

By learning problem specific HR synthesis models, our 3D MRI CNN strategy outperforms the naïve baseline up-sampling, quantitatively improving the

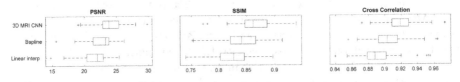

Fig. 3. PSNR, SSIM and Cross Correlation metrics for 45 LR image stacks with voxel spacing $(2.50 \times 2.50 \times 1.25)$ mm that are upsampled ×2 in-plane (X, Y) and compared to ground-truth image stacks $(1.25 \times 1.25 \times 1.25)$ mm using Linear, B-Spline, 3D MRI CNN methods.

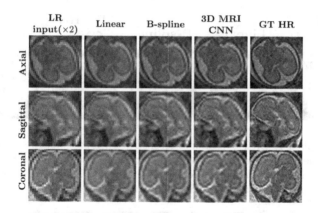

Fig. 4. Orthogonal fetal MRI stacks showing in-plane stack axes per row. Low resolution input (left) is upsampled by two baselines (col *Linear*, *B-spline*) and our learning based approach (col *3D MRI CNN*) *cf.* ground-truth (GT) HR imagery. The learning based 3D MRI CNN, with modality specific priors, provides improved high frequency signal components *cf.* baselines.

quality of the inferred HR imagery. Figure 4 exhibits an example of qualitative improvement in orthogonal fetal MRI test-stack axes.

We additionally perform preliminary experiments towards integrating network-based SR components more tightly with an SVR pipeline by investigating the ability of the network to upsample LR voxel intensities that result from an initial volume reconstruction iteration. Successful integration of an iterative (learning-based) SR and volume reconstruction loop will facilitate the well understood mutual benefits of reduced-motion SR input and improved input fidelity for the motion correction task. Qualitative comparison of (×4) LR volume-reconstructed input and resulting upsampled results are found in Fig. 5. The benefit of learning the upsampling with modality specific data can be observed to manifest as sharper edge gradients and improved high frequency signal components. The visual quality gap between the baselines and our method can be seen to widen as the prior information required to successfully upsample at larger factors make the task more challenging.

Volume Reconstruction Improvement: In our third experiment we evaluate SVR performance using LR input stacks, upsampled by the considered strategies, before initiating the volume reconstruction task. We additionally perform SVR reconstruction with original HR imagery to provide the "ground-truth" reference brain volumes. Employing the three quality metrics, introduced previously, we evaluate how well super-resolved LR stack reconstructions correspond to the reconstructions due to original high, in-plane, resolution imagery. Table 1 reports PSNR, SSIM and cross-correlation metrics for volume comparison (SR strategy with respect to "ground-truth" volume) for the 13 patients that define the MRI stack test set. Super-resolving the LR input data with the proposed learning based approach can be observed to facilitate reconstruction improvement,

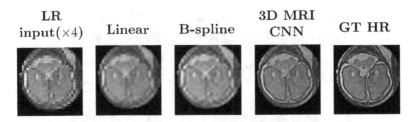

Fig. 5. SR applied to LR (×4) volume reconstructed input. Benefits of learning the specific non-linearities to recover sharp edge gradients and improved high frequency signal components of the modality become more evident *cf.* baselines as the amount of information required to upsample-successfully increases.

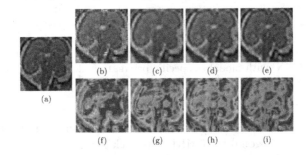

Fig. 6. (a) 2D slice through a fetal brain reconstruction, resulting from HR input-imagery. Attempting similar reconstruction from faster to acquire LR imagery, at half the in-plane resolution, results in highly degraded visual reconstruction quality (b) and gross DSSIM disparity (*ie.* red heatmap regions) (f) with respect to the HR reconstruction. Naïve up-sampling (×2) of the LR in-plane input prior to reconstruction, with linear interpolation or B-splines, result in over-smoothed input. Loss of sharp gradient information and input-image fidelity can be seen to propagate to the respective reconstructions (c), (d) and disparity, with regard to the HR reconstruction, remains high (g), (h). Our 3D MRI CNN upsampling affords input closer to the original HR imagery and results in improved reconstructions (e) and reduced DSSIM (i) with visibly cooler heatmap regions (standard *jet* color scale). (Color figure online)

across the investigated metrics. Visual evidence supporting this claim is found in Fig. 6 (best viewed in color). Figure 6 displays 2D slices of patient fetal brain reconstructions resulting from the original HR input-imagery (far left) and identically spatially-located slices (a) resulting from (b) LR imagery (half the in-plane resolution), (c-d) input using naïve up-sampling strategies and (e) our 3D MRI CNN upsampling. Corresponding Structural Dissimilarity (DSSIM) error heatmaps (second row) provide improved visual spatial congruence between HR ground-truth and our method, supporting the claim that utilizing sensor specific priors is of marked benefit for the task of MRI fetal brain reconstruction from LR imagery.

Table 1. PSNR, SSIM and Cross-correlation evaluating disparity between reconstructed volumes using upsampled LR input (Linear, B-Spline, 3D MRI CNN) and ground-truth volumes.

Upsample	PSNR *[dB]*	SSIM	Cross-correlation
No upsample	18.466 ± 1.88	0.534 ± 0.15	0.699 ± 0.12
Linear	19.268 ± 1.14	0.665 ± 0.08	0.815 ± 0.06
B-Spline	19.985 ± 1.52	0.698 ± 0.12	0.836 ± 0.08
3D MRI CNN	**21.715 ± 1.84**	**0.779 ± 0.10**	**0.885 ± 0.07**

5 Discussion and Conclusion

We introduce a 3D MRI CNN to upsample low resolution MR data prior to performing volumetric motion compensation and SVR reconstruction. Our method produces upsampled images and uses them to reconstruct volumetric fetal brain representations that quantitatively outperform on reconstruction tasks that utilise conventional upscaling methods. This contribution helps to address the well-understood image resolution challenge in fetal brain MRI. Analysis of accuracy metrics, assessing upsampling quality, exhibit a mean PSNR increase of 1.25 dB. Furthermore, when utilizing the upsampled imagery as SVR input, reconstructed fetal brain volumes show improvements of up to 1.73 dB over the provided baseline. In addition to quality improvement, 3D MRI CNN upsampling provides a computationally efficient approach affording an ability to initially image at lower resolutions, with a shorter acquisition time, thus provides faster and safer scanning for high-risk patients like pregnant women.

The current work has implicitly provided evidence that the method learns the PSF of the investigated MRI data well. In future it would be valuable to investigate this further, explicitly. Real-world LR/HR samples, acquired from scanners at differing resolutions, would allow quantitative evaluation of the ability to reconstruct physical scanner PSF and would further allow investigation of a model's ability to generalise to the reconstruction of PSFs not explicitly seen at training time. Further to this; the current work only investigates a single problem instance under one image modality. Future work will look to investigate the generalisability of the proposed framework to additional problem domains.

References

1. Borman, S., et al.: Super-resolution from image sequences-a review. In: Midwest Symposium on Circuits and Systems, pp. 374–378. IEEE (1998)
2. Çiçek, Ö., Abdulkadir, A., Lienkamp, S.S., Brox, T., Ronneberger, O.: 3D U-Net: learning dense volumetric segmentation from sparse annotation. In: Ourselin, S., Joskowicz, L., Sabuncu, M.R., Unal, G., Wells, W. (eds.) MICCAI 2016. LNCS, vol. 9901, pp. 424–432. Springer, Cham (2016). doi:10.1007/978-3-319-46723-8_49
3. Dong, C., Deng, Y., Loy, C.C., Tang, X.: Compression artifacts reduction by a deep convolutional network, pp. 576–584, December 2015

4. Dong, C., et al.: Image super-resolution using deep convolutional networks. IEEE Trans. PAMI **38**(2), 295–307 (2016)

5. Gholipour, A., et al.: Robust super-resolution volume reconstruction from slice acquisitions: application to fetal brain MRI. TMI **29**(10), 1739–1758 (2010)

6. Greenspan, H.: Super-resolution in medical imaging. Comput. J. **52**(1), 43–63 (2009)

7. Jia, Y., He, Z., Gholipour, A., Warfield, S.K.: Single anisotropic 3-D MR image upsampling via overcomplete dictionary trained from in-plane high resolution slices. IEEE J. Biomed. Health Inf. **20**(6), 1552–1561 (2016)

8. Kainz, B., et al.: Fast volume reconstruction from motion corrupted stacks of 2D slices. Trans. Med. Imag. **34**(9), 1901–1913 (2015)

9. Kamnitsas, K., Ferrante, E., Parisot, S., Ledig, C., Nori, A.V., Criminisi, A., Rueckert, D., Glocker, B.: DeepMedic for brain tumor segmentation. In: Crimi, A., Menze, B., Maier, O., Reyes, M., Winzeck, S., Handels, H. (eds.) Brain-Les 2016. LNCS, vol. 10154, pp. 138–149. Springer, Cham (2016). doi:10.1007/978-3-319-55524-9_14

10. Kim, K., et al.: Intersection based motion correction of multislice MRI for 3-D in utero fetal brain image formation. Trans. Med. Imag. **29**(1), 146–158 (2010)

11. Kuklisova-Murgasova, M., Quaghebeur, G., Rutherford, M.A., Hajnal, J.V., Schnabel, J.A.: Reconstruction of fetal brain MRI with intensity matching and complete outlier removal. Med. Image Anal. **16**(8), 1550–1560 (2012)

12. Ledig, C., et al.: Photo-realistic single image super-resolution using a generative adversarial network. In: Computer Vision and Pattern Recognition (CVPR) (2017)

13. Manjón, J.V., Coupé, P., Buades, A., Fonov, V., Collins, D.L., Robles, M.: Nonlocal MRI upsampling. Med. Image Anal. **14**(6), 784–792 (2010)

14. Nasrollahi, K., et al.: Super-resolution: a comprehensive survey. Mach. Vis. Appl. **25**(6), 1423–1468 (2014)

15. Oktay, O., et al.: Multi-input cardiac image super-resolution using convolutional neural networks. In: Ourselin, S., Joskowicz, L., Sabuncu, M.R., Unal, G., Wells, W. (eds.) MICCAI 2016. LNCS, vol. 9902, pp. 246–254. Springer, Cham (2016). doi:10.1007/978-3-319-46726-9_29

16. Rousseau, F., Kim, K., Studholme, C., Koob, M., Dietemann, J.-L.: On super-resolution for fetal brain MRI. In: Jiang, T., Navab, N., Pluim, J.P.W., Viergever, M.A. (eds.) MICCAI 2010. LNCS, vol. 6362, pp. 355–362. Springer, Heidelberg (2010). doi:10.1007/978-3-642-15745-5_44

17. Rousseau, F., et al.: Registration-based approach for reconstruction of high-resolution in utero fetal MR brain images. Acad. Radiol. **13**(9), 1072–1081 (2006)

18. Rousseau, F., et al.: BTK: an open-source toolkit for fetal brain MR image processing. Comput. Methods Programs Biomed. **109**(1), 65–73 (2013)

19. Shi, W., Caballero, J., Huszár, F., Totz, J., Aitken, A.P., Bishop, R., Rueckert, D., Wang, Z.: Real-time single image and video super-resolution using an efficient sub-pixel convolutional neural network, pp. 1874–1883 (2016)

20. Simonyan, K., et al.: very deep convolutional networks for large-scale image recognition. arXiv:1409.1556 abs/1409.1556 (2014)

21. Tourbier, S., Bresson, X., Hagmann, P., Thiran, J.P., Meuli, R., Cuadra, M.B.: An efficient total variation algorithm for super-resolution in fetal brain MRI with adaptive regularization. NeuroImage **118**, 584–597 (2015)

Reconstruction of 3D Cardiac MR Images from 2D Slices Using Directional Total Variation

Nicolas Basty[1]([✉]), Darryl McClymont[2], Irvin Teh[2,3], Jürgen E. Schneider[2,3], and Vicente Grau[1]

[1] Department of Engineering Science, Institute of Biomedical Engineering,
University of Oxford, Oxford, UK
nicolas.basty@eng.ox.ac.uk
[2] Division of Cardiovascular Medicine, Radcliffe Department of Medicine,
University of Oxford, Oxford, UK
[3] Leeds Institute of Cardiovascular and Metabolic Medicine,
University of Leeds, Leeds, UK

Abstract. Cardiac MRI allows for the acquisition of high resolution images of the heart. Long acquisition times of MRI make it impractical to image the full heart in 3D at high resolution. As a result, multiple 2D images are commonly acquired with a slice thickness greater than the in-plane resolution. One way of achieving isotropic high-resolution images is to apply post-processing techniques such as super-resolution to produce high resolution images from low resolution input. We use short-axis stacks as well as orthogonal long-axis views in a super-resolution framework, constraining the reconstruction using the contrast independent directional total variation algorithm to produce a high resolution 3D reconstruction with isotropic resolution. The 3D reconstruction retains the contrast of the short-axis stack, but incorporates the edge information from both the short-axis and the long-axis stacks. Results show improved reconstructions, with a segmentation voxel misclassification rate of 3.51% as opposed to 4.27% using linear interpolation.

Keywords: 3D image reconstruction · Super-resolution · Cardiac MRI · Regularisation · Directional total variation

1 Introduction

Magnetic Resonance Imaging (MRI) is a non-ionising and non-invasive imaging method exhibiting particularly good soft tissue contrast. It provides structural as well as functional information, and it is taken as gold standard for soft tissue imaging notably for vital organs such as the brain and the heart. In a clinical setting, patient motion from breathing, cardiac motion as well as long acquisition times restrict imaging from being performed at full isotropic 3D high resolution routinely. As a consequence, 2D slices with highly anisotropic voxels are acquired. The standard clinical protocol is to image a set of stacked parallel short-axis (SA) images and a smaller number of long-axis (LA) views orthogonal to the SA stack

© Springer International Publishing AG 2017
M.J. Cardoso et al. (Eds.): CMMI/RAMBO/SWITCH 2017, LNCS 10555, pp. 127–135, 2017.
DOI: 10.1007/978-3-319-67564-0_13

covering most of the heart. 2D low resolution (LR) slices are typically acquired with in-plane pixel size of 1–2 mm and slice thickness of 6–10 mm with a small slice gap of 2–4 mm [1]. SA image stacks often fail to capture the apex or the base of the heart appropriately, and data for those essential features is only contained in the LA slices. In practice, one 4-chamber view and one 2-chamber view are acquired, making it very imbalanced between numbers of SA and LA acquisitions. However, this choice of orientation is not made with the aim of reconstructing a 3D volume.

Methods for improving image quality may occur at different points along the image reconstruction pipeline. For example, compressed sensing algorithms work with the acquired k-space data, reconstructing images using sparse modelling. This serves to decrease imaging time whilst still giving adequate image quality [2]. The technique has been successfully applied to dynamic 2D CMR reconstructions [3]. Other algorithms operate after images have been reconstructed, performing de-noising, super-resolution or other post-processing techniques. The proposed algorithm falls into the latter category. Super-resolution in MRI has first been described in [4], in which a reconstruction algorithm is applied on acquisitions with small shifts in the slice selection direction, giving improved resolution and edge definition. In super-resolution MRI reconstruction, the imaging process is generally modelled as follows: A real ground truth object $\mathbf{G}$ is imaged by a process resulting in an image, $\mathbf{X}$. This is modelled by applying a transformation $\mathbf{T}$ and additive gaussian noise n $\mathbf{X} = \mathbf{TG} + n$. The operator $\mathbf{T}$ is defined as a combination of geometric transformations, convolution with a point-spread function, which is often a Gaussian kernel, and downsampling [5]. Having defined an acquisition model, the image reconstruction process can be posed as an ill-conditioned inverse problem. In addition to the data consistency term, different regularisers R have been applied [6,7]. Such regularisers control features of the reconstructions such as the magnitude of edges and degree of smoothness, and allow ill-conditioned problems to be solved as follows:

$$\mathbf{Y} = \min_{Y} \sum_{i=1}^{N} ||\mathbf{T}_i \mathbf{Y} - \mathbf{x}_i||^2 + \lambda R \tag{1}$$

Where $\mathbf{Y}$ is the reconstruction, N 2D slices are used, and λ determines the weighting of the regularisation term.

The feasibility of such super-resolution methods was shown by Plenge et al. [8], in which they compared iterative back-projection, algebraic reconstruction and regularised least squares algorithms on phantoms and in vivo MRI. In [7,9], a Laplacian regulariser is applied to control the high spatial frequencies on reconstruction of small bird and full body mouse MRI images, giving good qualitative results and outperforming standard interpolation techniques. However, as opposed to sparse sampled cardiac MRI, most of the imaging volume is sampled in those studies.

Total variation is another popular regulariser with edge-preserving and convex characteristics, and has especially been used for de-noising [10]. It has also been applied to super-resolution and compressed sensing of MRI data as a regulariser [11]. An added difficulty in cardiac MRI are the differences in intensity and contrast between SA and LA acquisitions occurring because of different imaging protocols and sequence timings. Thus, any reconstruction algorithm aiming to reconstruct images using information from both the SA and LA images must be contrast independent. Directional total variation (dTV) is a recently introduced approach for reconstructing images using a reference image with the same structure but different contrast. In a study by Ehrhardt *et al.* [12] 2D dTV is used to combine information from brain MRI with different T1 and T2 weightings. It uses one image and its structural information as a reference for the dTV to guide the reconstruction of the other. A different regulariser which has been applied to super-resolution of CMR is the Beltrami regularisation [13] in which they solve Eq. (1) using three sets of image stacks covering the whole left ventricle in the SA, horizonal LA and vertical LA orientations. Limitations of this work are that the slice protocol used does not reflect clinical practice as the number of slices is a lot higher, and it does not address differences in contrast between SA and LA. Recent studies such as work by Oktay *et al.* [14] have focused on the use of Convolutional Neural Networks for super-resolution of CMR and shown great promise. However, methods based on machine learning make the assumption that testing data is well represented by the training data, which may not hold in pathological cases.

In this work, we address the problem of reconstructing 3D images from a stack of 2D slices in both SA and LA orientations, in a contrast-independent manner using the directional total variation regulariser. This allows a reconstructed image with the contrast of the short-axis images but with the additional structural information of the LA images.

2 Materials and Methods

2.1 Image Acquisition

Experimental investigations conformed to the UK Home Office guidance on the Operations of Animals (Scientific Procedures) Act 1986 and were approved by the University of Oxford ethical review board. One heart was excised from a female Sprague-Dawley rat during terminal anaesthesia, fixed then embedded in 1% agarose gel, and imaged on a 9.4 T preclinical MRI scanner (Agilent, CA, USA). A single 3D gradient echo image was acquired: FOV = 25.6 × 25.6 × 25.6 mm, acquisition matrix = 384 × 384 × 384, TR = 200 ms, TE = 4 ms, flip angle = 60°, scan time = 8.2 h. LR 2D slices $\mathbf{X}$: FOV = 25.6 × 25.6 mm, acquisition matrix = 128 × 128, in-plane resolution = 0.2 mm, slice thickness = 1 mm were synthetically generated from the 3D image $\mathbf{Y}$ using the sampling function $\mathbf{T}$, such that $\mathbf{X}_i = \mathbf{T}_i \mathbf{Y}$. The sampling function differs to the ones generally used in the literature by working in k-space. Instead of averaging points in image space, the Fourier transform of $\mathbf{Y}$ is truncated in k-space, after rotation of the

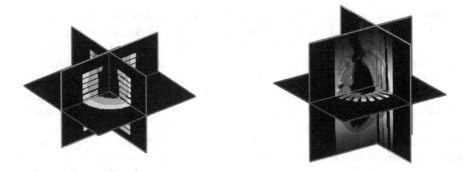

Fig. 1. LHS: cut through 3D view of 11 SA in 3D space. The blue plane is aligned with the SA while the red and green planes are aligned with the LA. RHS: cut through 3D view of 11 LA in 3D space. The LA slices have noticeably different contrast than the SA slices. (Color figure online)

3D image. The image is rotated such that the in-plane view corresponds to the orientation of the slice to be synthetised. The LA images were synthetised after applying a histogram shift to the ground truth 3D volume, to ensure the LR SA, and LA images have different contrast. This is visible in Fig. 1.

2.2 Super-Resolution Algorithm

We formulate the problem by simultaneously solving the following

$$\mathbf{Y}_{SA}^* = \arg\min_{\mathbf{Y}_{SA}} \sum_{i=1}^{n_{SA}} ||\mathbf{T}_i\mathbf{Y}_{SA} - \mathbf{X}_i||_2^2 + \lambda J(\mathbf{Y}_{SA}, \mathbf{Y}_{LA}) \tag{2}$$

$$\mathbf{Y}_{LA}^* = \arg\min_{\mathbf{Y}_{LA}} \sum_{j=1}^{n_{LA}} ||\mathbf{T}_j\mathbf{Y}_{LA} - \mathbf{X}_j||_2^2 + \lambda J(\mathbf{Y}_{LA}, \mathbf{Y}_{SA}) \tag{3}$$

In both (2) and (3), the first term in the problem is related to data accuracy, ensuring that the current estimate does not deviate too much from the 2D LR image $\mathbf{X}_i$ which are the ground truth measurements. The second term sets a constraint using the directional total variation of the image. It pushes the first term in J towards being smooth whilst using the structural information of the second term in J as a reference. λ is a weight adjusting the contribution of the directional total variation term. The 3D directional total variation constraint J applied to image $\mathbf{A}$ with reference image $\mathbf{B}$ is defined as follows [12]:

$$J(\mathbf{A}, \mathbf{B}) = \sum_{n=1}^{3} |D_n \nabla \mathbf{A}_n| \tag{4}$$

where matrix field $D_n \in \mathbb{M}^3 = 1 - \xi_n \xi_n^*$ and $\xi_n := \frac{\nabla B_n}{|\nabla B_n|_\eta}$. The tuning parameter η relates to the size of the edges in reference image $\mathbf{B}$. Equations (2) and (3) were simultaneously solved using nonlinear conjugate gradient optimisation [15], in which one step towards the minimum in both Eqs. (2) and (3) was taken during each iteration. The image $\mathbf{Y}_{SA}$ was initialised by putting the LR SA slices into their respective orientations in a 3D matrix with isotropic spacing matching the LR in-plane resolution. The gaps between slices are filled by linear interpolation for a fairer comparison than just using nearest neighbor. $\mathbf{Y}_{LA}$ is initialised in similar fashion, by putting the LR LA slices into a 3D matrix and filling the gaps using nearest neighbour interpolation. Voxels where the LA slices overlap are averaged. Nonlinear conjugate gradient method alternates between iterations as to which image to reconstruct of to use as a reference for the dTV. The λ parameter was empirically set to 0.5 and the η parameter was set to 0.05. Data consistency checks SA LR within the SA reconstruction, and LA LR within the LA reconstruction. The process is repeated until convergence. Results are shown on the SA reconstruction as the aim is to increase their through-plane resolution.

2.3 Validation

The 3D reconstructions will be validated against the HR ground truth image acquired for that purpose, using the Peak-Signal-to-Noise ratio (PSNR) which is widely used in image quality assessment because of its simplicity and clear physical meaning. However, this metric is often criticised for not matching visual quality. In addition, we evaluate the Dice score as well as voxel misclassification for segmentations of the Left Ventricular volume by binarising the images via simple thresholding and give a percentage of misclassified voxels. The contrast between the myocardium and the left ventricle is sufficient that the segmentation result is insensitive to minor changes in the threshold value. The experiment will be run using 11 SA and 11 LA slices covering most of the space, and then with a total number of 12 slices with different combinations of LA and SA acquisitions as to not use more slices than acquired in practice.

3 Results

Table 1 contains qualitative results for reconstructions using 3 different combinations of slices. The first one was chosen to resemble clinical acquisitions with a highly unbalanced number of SA and LA slices. The second one was chosen to balance them by taking an equal number of each orientation, and the third one was done to see if an increased number of LA slices is of benefit.

The result in Fig. 2 shows a cut in LA orientation through the final reconstruction, at an orientation not covered by one of the 11 ground truth LA slices, for a fair comparison. The synthetic slices cover most of the space and do not represent a real clinical scenario. In order for a more realistic approach, we chose

Table 1. Quantitative results: Dice score, Voxel misclassifications and Peak-Signal-to-Noise Ratio in the reconstruction and in the interpolated image.

	9 SA, 3 LA	6 LA, 6 SA	3 SA, 9 LA
Dice score (Reconstruction)	0.9690	0.9762	0.9629
Dice score (Interpolation)	0.9742	0.9710	0.9426
Misclassification (Reconstruction)	4.45%	3.51%	5.37%
Misclassification (Interpolation)	3.70%	4.27%	8.18%
PSNR (Reconstruction)	13.52 dB	14.59 dB	12.69 dB
PSNR (Interpolation)	14.31 dB	13.69 dB	10.08 dB

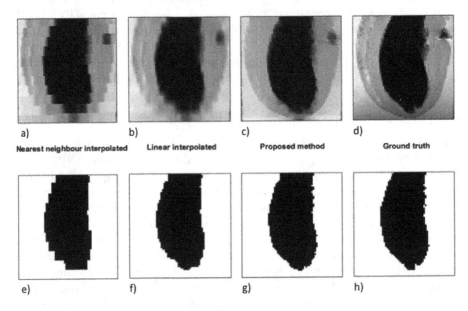

Fig. 2. (a) 11 SA slices in 3D space with nearest neighbour interpolation (b) Initialisation achieved by linear interpolation between 11 SA slices, (c) Reconstruction using the framework aided by 11 SA and 11 LA slices (d) Ground truth (e) Segmentation of nearest neighbour (f) Segmentation of interpolation image, (g) Segmentation of reconstruction (h) Segmentation of ground truth

to use 12 synthetic acquisitions - 6 LA and 6 SA. The more clinically used combination of approximately 10 SA and 2 LA leaves space very under-sampled for through plane detail, especially around the apex and base. Similarly to Fig. 2, the result in Fig. 3 shows a cut in LA orientation through the final reconstruction, at an orientation not covered by one of the 6 ground truth LA slices.

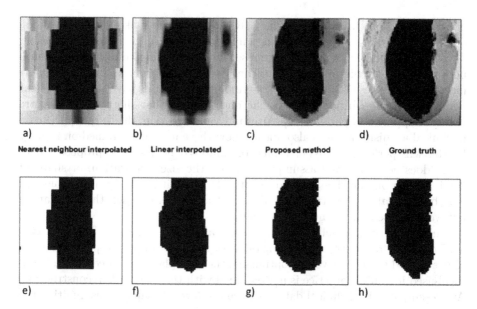

Fig. 3. (a) 6 SA slices in 3D space with nearest neighbour interpolation (b) Initialisation achieved by linear interpolation between 6 SA slices, (c) Reconstruction using the framework aided by 6 SA and 6 LA slices (d) Ground truth (e) Segmentation of nearest neighbour (f) Segmentation of interpolation image, (g) Segmentation of reconstruction, (h) Segmentation of ground truth

4   Discussion and Conclusion

The reconstruction using 9 SA and 3 LA slices does not show improvements with respect to interpolation on any of the metrics that were applied (cf. Table 1), whereas the reconstruction using 3 SA and 9 LA slices does show improvements in the metrics, but starting off with worse quantitative results on the initialisation. This highlights our finding that the slice protocol followed in clinical practice is not ideal for 3D reconstruction, and that increasing the number of LA slices improves the reconstruction. Balancing the number of LA and SA slices shows improvements which outperform the interpolation.

This work has addressed the problem of combining structural information from long-axis images to improve the generation of 3D volumes from short-axis images. Accurate 3D volumes are required for the generation of meshes for mechanical models as well as other applications such as measuring cardiac volumes or estimating ejection fractions.

There are some limitations to this study. The algorithm assumes a preprocessing step of SA-LA registration, and any inaccuracies in this step will be propagated into the image reconstruction. Furthermore, as it is based on total variation, regions outside the sampled planes will typically be as smooth as possible (i.e. the image in-painting is extremely crude). It is therefore crucial that as much of the heart as possible is imaged by at least one plane, which is not currently done in clinical cardiac MRI. Between the spokes of the LA slices, only the SA is driving the reconstruction and is highly sensitive to initialisation.

Unlike a number of recently proposed methods using convolutional neural networks [14,16], the proposed algorithm does not incorporate any prior information. While these CNN based super-resolution methods have shown excellent performance, the cardiac MRI specific ones assume that short-axis stacks are non-overlapping and parallel [17]. After motion correction, this is rarely the case in clinical acquisitions. It is also unclear how these networks, trained on healthy hearts, will perform on hypertrophic or infarcted hearts. The proposed algorithm does not make any assumptions about the size, orientation, or shape of the heart, or on the slice selection protocol. Thus, it is widely applicable and may be preferable when training data is not available, or when the test data is not well represented by the training data.

Further work will include extending the algorithm to use all frames of cine MRI datasets, rather than operating on a static image. Improved performance is also expected to be achieved by optimising the slice planning, since the slice protocol used in clinical practice is not designed with the aim of 3D reconstruction. At present, standard clinical datasets have too few LA acquisitions, limiting the algorithm's performance.

Acknowledgments. NMB acknowledges the support of the RCUK Digital Economy Programme grant number EP/G036861/1 (Oxford Centre for Doctoral Training in Healthcare Innovation). This work was supported by the British Heart Foundation (BHF) [grant numbers PG/13/33/30210, RG/13/8/30266, FS/11/50/29038 and NH/13/30238], the Engineering and Physical Sciences Research Council [grant number EP/J013250/1], and the BHF Centre for Research Excellence [grant number RE/13/1/30181. The authors acknowledge a Wellcome Trust Core Award [grant number 090532/Z/09/Z].

References

1. Bogaert, J., Dymarkowski, S., Taylor, A.M.: Clinical Cardiac MRI. Taylor & Francis US (2005)
2. Lustig, M., Donoho, D., Pauly, J.M.: Sparse MRI: the application of compressed sensing for rapid MR imaging. Magn. Reson. Med. **58**(6), 1182–1195 (2007)
3. Caballero, J., Price, A.N., Rueckert, D., Hajnal, J.V.: Dictionary learning and time sparsity for dynamic MR data reconstruction. IEEE Trans. Med. Imaging **33**(4), 979–94 (2014)
4. Greenspan, H., Oz, G., Kiryati, N., Peled, S.: MRI inter-slice reconstruction using super-resolution. Magn. Reson. Imaging **20**(5), 437–446 (2002)
5. Van Reeth, E., Tham, I.: Superresolution in magnetic resonance imaging: a review. Concepts Magn. Reson. Part A **40A**(6), 306–325 (2012)
6. Woo, J., Murano, E., Stone, M., Prince, J.: Reconstruction of high resolution tongue volumes from MRI. IEEE Trans. Biomed. Eng. **59**(12), 1–1 (2012)
7. Poot, D.H.J., Meir, V., Sijbers, J.: General and efficient super-resolution method for multi-slice MRI. In: Jiang, T., Navab, N., Pluim, J.P.W., Viergever, M.A. (eds.) MICCAI 2010. LNCS, vol. 6361, pp. 615–622. Springer, Heidelberg (2010). doi:10. 1007/978-3-642-15705-9_75

8. Plenge, E., Poot, D.H.J., Bernsen, M., Kotek, G., Houston, G., Wielopolski, P., Van Der Weerd, L., Niessen, W.J., Meijering, E.: Super-resolution methods in MRI: can they improve the trade-off between resolution, signal-to-noise ratio, and acquisition time? Magn. Reson. Med. **68**(6), 1983–1993 (2012)

9. Khmelinskii, A., Plenge, E., Kok, P., Dzyubachyk, O., Poot, D.H.J., Suidgeest, E., Botha, C.P., Niessen, W.J., van der Weerd, L., Meijering, E., et al.: Super-resolution reconstruction of whole-body MRI mouse data: an interactive approach. In: 2012 9th IEEE International Symposium on Biomedical Imaging (ISBI), pp. 1723–1726. IEEE (2012)

10. Rudin, L.I., Osher, S., Fatemi, E.: Nonlinear total variation based noise removal algorithms. Physica D **60**(1–4), 259–268 (1992)

11. Joshi, S.H., Marquina, A., Osher, S.J., Dinov, I., Van Horn, J.D., Toga, A.W.: MRI resolution enhancement using total variation regularization. In: 2009 IEEE International Symposium on Biomedical Imaging: From Nano to Macro, ISBI 2009, pp. 161–164. IEEE (2009)

12. Ehrhardt, M.J., Betcke, M.M.: Multicontrast MRI reconstruction with structure-guided total variation. SIAM J. Imaging Sci. **9**(3), 1084–1106 (2016)

13. Odille, F., Bustin, A., Chen, B., Vuissoz, P.-A., Felblinger, J.: Motion-corrected, super-resolution reconstruction for high-resolution 3D cardiac cine MRI. In: Navab, N., Hornegger, J., Wells, W.M., Frangi, A.F. (eds.) MICCAI 2015. LNCS, vol. 9351, pp. 435–442. Springer, Cham (2015). doi:10.1007/978-3-319-24574-4_52

14. Oktay, O., et al.: Multi-input cardiac image super-resolution using convolutional neural networks. In: Ourselin, S., Joskowicz, L., Sabuncu, M.R., Unal, G., Wells, W. (eds.) MICCAI 2016. LNCS, vol. 9902, pp. 246–254. Springer, Cham (2016). doi:10.1007/978-3-319-46726-9_29

15. Shewchuk, J.R.: An introduction to the conjugate gradient method without the agonizing pain (1994)

16. Dong, C., Loy, C.C., He, K., Tang, X.: Learning a deep convolutional network for image super-resolution. In: Fleet, D., Pajdla, T., Schiele, B., Tuytelaars, T. (eds.) ECCV 2014. LNCS, vol. 8692, pp. 184–199. Springer, Cham (2014). doi:10.1007/978-3-319-10593-2_13

17. Oktay, O., Ferrante, E., Kamnitsas, K., Heinrich, M., Bai, W., Caballero, J., Guerrero, R., Cook, S., de Marvao, A., O'Regan, D., et al.: Anatomically constrained neural networks (ACNN): application to cardiac image enhancement and segmentation. arXiv preprint arXiv:1705.08302 (2017)

An Efficient Multi-resolution Reconstruction Scheme with Motion Compensation for 5D Free-Breathing Whole-Heart MRI

Rosa-María Menchón-Lara[1]([✉]), Javier Royuela-del-Val[1],
Alejandro Godino-Moya[1], Lucilio Cordero-Grande[2],
Federico Simmross-Wattenberg[1], Marcos Martín-Fernández[1],
and Carlos Alberola-López[1]

[1] Image Processing Lab, University of Valladolid, Valladolid, Spain
rmenchon@lpi.tel.uva.es
[2] Department of Biomedical Engineering, King's College London, London, UK

Abstract. In this work, we propose a novel approach for the reconstruction of 3D isotropic, free-breathing cardiac cine MRI with 100% data efficiency. The main components are a continuous 3D Golden radial k-space data acquisition, a robust groupwise cardio-respiratory motion estimation technique and a multiresolution strategy introduced in a previously proposed compressed sensing reconstruction scheme. Initial results on simulated data show better reconstruction quality than the non-motion compensated counterpart and reduced reconstruction times with respect to a single-resolution procedure for equivalent acceleration factors ranging 24.38 to 34.8.

1 Introduction

Cardiovascular diseases (CVDs) are the first cause of death, with 17.5 million estimated deaths in 2012 (about 31% of all deceases in the world). As for detection and follow up of CVDs, magnetic resonance imaging (MRI) has become the reference imaging modality in anatomic and functional heart studies due to its high contrast and spatiotemporal resolution.

However, MRI is a slow technique in terms of acquisition time and it is also highly sensitive to motion of the inspected structures. Specifically, motion induced by both the natural heart motion as well as patient breathing translate itself in artifacted images, a fact that constitutes one of the major challenges, still today, in cine cardiac MRI.

Cine MRI lets the practitioner visualize heart motion along the whole cardiac cycle, which, in turn, allows the physician to calculate descriptive parameters of both the function and the anatomy as well as to detect and diagnose contractility anomalies. In a conventional cine examination, a set of two-dimensional slices covering the full cardiac volume (or, at least, the left ventricle) is obtained. To mitigate the effect of motion in acquisition, current clinical practice either makes use of breath hold procedures or navigators that trigger image acquisition

© Springer International Publishing AG 2017
M.J. Cardoso et al. (Eds.): CMMI/RAMBO/SWITCH 2017, LNCS 10555, pp. 136–145, 2017.
DOI: 10.1007/978-3-319-67564-0_14

intervals at certain positions of the diaphragm along the respiratory cycle; the two processes, however, are highly inefficient since a large fraction of the time spent by the patient within the magnet is not effective acquisition time. The final result is a set of 2D+t dynamic images whose spacing is typically several times higher than the intra-slice resolution (e.g., 8 mm inter-slice vs. 2 mm intra-slice). This remarked anisotropy has an additional implication: due to the complex orientation of the heart in the thoracic cavity, a previous planification stage is mandatory, in which the orientation planes of the image are carefully chosen to match the principal axes of the heart. 3D approaches naturally avoid these problems.

In order to speed up the acquisition procedure, compressed sensing (CS) techniques have been proposed and they are now relatively mature. These techniques basically consist in drastically subsampling k-space. Then, the reconstruction procedure is solved by constrained optimization procedures based on the assumption that natural images are sparse in some transformed domain.

MRI sparse reconstruction, when it is applied to dynamic modalities, can benefit from the high redundancy level typically found along the temporal dimension of the image. As an example, in cine, intensity variations of a voxel in time will be mainly due to the motion of cardiac structures (ideally, if a material point is perfectly tracked, intensity should be constant). Motion effects on the sparse representations have already been addressed in the literature [1,7,8,11,15,16]. In the cited methods, the authors share the idea that a sparser representation can be obtained when information about the motion present in the image is introduced in the sparsifying transform, enabling higher acceleration factors.

In order to increase the scan efficiency, several techniques have been proposed [4,5,14]; these techniques do not restrict data acquisition to certain respiratory states but data are continuously acquired following a radial trajectory in the k-space without respiratory gating. Cardiac and respiratory signals can be acquired simultaneously or estimated from the acquired data. These two signals are used to bin the data into several respiratory and cardiac states according to the breathing position and cardiac phase at which they were acquired. Images are then reconstructed imposing spatio-temporal smoothness constraints.

In this paper, we show that better results can be obtained by incorporating motion estimation (ME) and compensation (MC) methods in the optimization procedure for 3D isotropic whole-heart free-breathing cine reconstruction. Motion is estimated by means of a groupwise nonrigid registration paradigm, which has already been used for the 2D case by the authors [16]. For the 3D case, computational load is much higher so we have resorted to a multiresolution procedure, in which motion is estimated and images are reconstructed. Higher levels of the pyramid are then interpolated and serve as the starting point of the immediate lower level of the pyramid. Results indicate that this procedure better preserves edges and shows a better contrast than methods that do not incorporate this type of information in the reconstruction procedure. In summary, this paper proposes an extension of the XD-GRASP [6] reconstruction framework for free-breathing acquired data based on introducing a MC approach and a multi-resolution scheme.

2   Material and Methods

2.1   Compressed Sensing Reconstruction

The problem of MRI reconstruction under CS principle is defined as follows:

$$\underset{\mathbf{m}}{\text{argmin}} \, \|\boldsymbol{\Phi}\mathbf{m}\|_{l1} \text{ s.t. } \|\mathbf{y} - \mathbf{Em}\|_{l2}^2 < \epsilon \tag{1}$$

where $\mathbf{m}$ represents the image to reconstruct from the acquired undersampled k-t data ($\mathbf{y}$) and ϵ indicates the noise level in the acquisition. $\boldsymbol{\Phi}$ is the sparsifying transform, which is typically chosen to be the temporal Fourier transform or the temporal total variation. The encoding operator $\mathbf{E}$ models the acquisition process by applying spatial Fourier transforms followed by the data undersampling strategy. Moreover, in multicoil acquisitions, $\mathbf{E}$ also includes the multiplication by coil sensitivities [12]. Finally, the constrained problem in Eq. (1) can be reformulated as the following equivalent unconstrained optimization problem:

$$\underset{\mathbf{m}}{\text{argmin}} \frac{1}{2} \, \|\mathbf{y} - \mathbf{Em}\|_{l2}^2 + \lambda \, \|\boldsymbol{\Phi}\mathbf{m}\|_{l1} \tag{2}$$

where the parameter λ establishes a trade-off between data consistency and the sparsity of the solution.

2.2   Motion Compensated MRI Reconstruction

In CS with motion estimation and compensation (ME/MC), the operator $\boldsymbol{\Phi}$ is modified to include some knowledge about the specific motion of the structures being imaged. In particular, in groupwise (GW) CS [16], the authors propose a joint estimation and compensation of the motion in the whole image domain, and the optimization problem in Eq. (2) becomes

$$\underset{\mathbf{m}}{\text{argmin}} \frac{1}{2} \, \|\mathbf{y} - \mathbf{Em}\|_{l2}^2 + \lambda \, \|\boldsymbol{\Phi}\mathcal{T}_{\Theta}\mathbf{m}\|_{l1} \tag{3}$$

where $\mathcal{T}_{\Theta}$ is the GW-MC operator, a set of spatial deformations defined by the parameters Θ, that performs a mapping between each temporal instant in the dynamic image and a common reference motion state. Note that the motion in $\mathbf{m}$ is unknown a priori. Therefore, firstly, it is necessary to perform a regular CS reconstruction by solving Eq. (2).

Essentially, this motion estimation method consists on a GW registration method based on a B-spline deformation model with set of control points Θ. The registration metric is defined based on the variance of the intensity along time, and the control points that minimize its value are found as follows:

$$\underset{\Theta}{\text{argmin}} \left\| \sum_{n=1}^{N} \left(\mathcal{T}_{\Theta,n}\mathbf{m}_n - \frac{1}{N} \sum_{k=1}^{N} \mathcal{T}_{\Theta,k}\mathbf{m}_k \right) \right\|^2 + \mathcal{R}_{\Theta} \tag{4}$$

where n and k represent the time index, N is the total of temporal instants (number of images/volumes to reconstruct) and $\mathcal{R}_\Theta$ is an additional regularization term that encourages local invertibility of the deformations [3]. This regularization term is based on the Laplace operator and second order temporal derivatives of the deformation fields and it can be compactly expressed as follows:

$$\mathcal{R}_\Theta = \alpha \left\| \Delta \mathcal{T}_{\Theta,n} \right\|_2^2 + \beta \left\| \nabla_n^2 \mathcal{T}_{\Theta,n} \right\|_2^2 \tag{5}$$

2.3 Extra-Dimensinal (XD) MRI Reconstruction

A recently proposed approach for the reconstruction of free-breathing acquired data (XD-GRASP) [6] is based on the continuous acquisition of k-space data following a 3D Golden Radial trajectory [10] (Fig. 1a). Data are then distributed in different respiratory and cardiac phases (double binning process, Fig. 1b), which results in a 5D domain (k_x, k_y, k_z, respiratory phase and cardiac phase). This division is made in accordance with the respiratory and cardiac motion signals, with the approximately same number of spokes in each temporal frame.

The reconstruction is formulated as a CS problem in which sparsity along both temporal dimensions is simultaneously enforced:

$$\operatorname*{argmin}_{\mathbf{m}} \frac{1}{2} \left\| \mathbf{y} - \mathbf{E}\mathbf{m} \right\|_{l2}^2 + \lambda_c \left\| \nabla_c \mathbf{m} \right\|_{l1} + \lambda_r \left\| \nabla_r \mathbf{m} \right\|_{l1} \tag{6}$$

where ∇_c and ∇_r stand for the temporal differences along the cardiac and respiratory phases, respectively. As a result of the reconstruction, a set of 3D+t volumes is recovered, one for each respiratory state (Fig. 1c).

Since the data is divided into more motion states, less data is available for each of them, increasing the net acceleration factor consequently. Moreover, the size of the solution space is also increased, rising the computational cost.

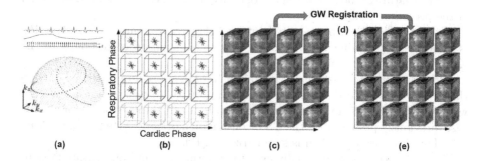

Fig. 1. Overview of the proposed reconstruction method: (a) data acquisition strategy: 3D golden radial sampling; (b) binned data: respiratory and cardiac phases; (c) initial CS reconstruction; (d) motion estimation by means of a GW registration method; (e) final MC-CS reconstruction.

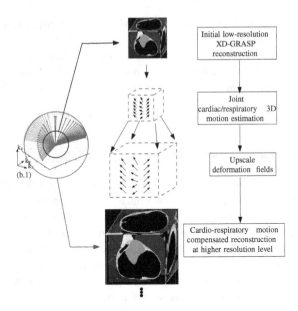

Fig. 2. Overview of the proposed multi-resolution scheme for MC-XD MRI reconstruction. For the low resolution reconstruction only the central portion of k-space data is used (blue circle). While for the upper resolution level resolution, scaled deformation fields and all acquired k-space data (red circle) are used. (Color figure online)

2.4   Multi-resolution Strategy for MC-XD MRI Reconstruction

In this work, we propose to extend the XD scheme in two ways: (1) by introducing a MC approach in which both the cardiac and respiratory motions are considered during reconstruction and (2) by introducing a multi-resolution approach in which the nature of the radial k-space data acquisition is exploited. A description of the procedure follows.

Once the data has been sorted into a 5D space, an initial reconstruction is performed by solving Eq. (6), see Fig. 1c. This solution corresponds to the XD-GRASP method [5,6].

Once an initial reconstruction is available, a ME procedure is carried out. To this end, we resort to the 3D extension of a group-wise registration algorithm, which provides robust motion estimation, both in and through-plane for the 3D case, previously proposed for the CS reconstruction of multi-slice 2D CINE MRI [16]. The estimation problem is summarized in Eq. (4).

The obtained results are finally used to perform a motion compensated reconstruction over the initial images (Fig. 1e), being possible to iterate over the last two steps to refine the results. MC-XD reconstruction can be formulated as:

$$\underset{\mathbf{m}}{\mathrm{argmin}} \frac{1}{2} \|\mathbf{y} - \mathbf{E}\mathbf{m}\|_{l2}^2 + \lambda \|\boldsymbol{\nabla}_{c,r} \mathcal{T}_{\Theta}^{c,r} \mathbf{m}\|_{l1} \tag{7}$$

where $\mathcal{T}_\Theta^{c,r}$ is the MC operator that compensates both for cardiac and respiratory motions and $\nabla_{c,r}$ calculates the gradient along both temporal dimensions.

Computational efficiency can be highly improved by means of the multiresolution algorithm we propose in this work, a graphical sketch of which is shown in Fig. 2. In particular, we propose to perform the aforementioned process at minimal spatial resolution, that is, to obtain the initial reconstruction (XD-GRASP) at low resolution by using only the central portion of the k-space data, and to apply the motion estimation approach (3D GW registration) at this level. To this end we exploit the fact that, in radial trajectories, the central region of the k-space is sampled much more densely that the high frequency domain. In this situation, the resulting acceleration factor at the low resolution level is much lower than the original one, leading to a better posed reconstruction problem with lower computational demand.

Then, by means of an upscaling procedure, both initial images and deformation fields are interpolated to a higher resolution level. A cubic 3D interpolation is applied for the image upscaling. While for the registration results, the set of control points is scaled to recalculate the deformation fields. The obtained results are then used as the starting point to perform the MC reconstruction in the following upper level.

2.5   Data and Experiments Description

The proposed strategy has been tested on synthetic data generated by a numerical phantom that provides detailed internal anatomy and realistic cardiorespiratory deformation models [13,18]. A bSSFP acquisition was simulated in free-breathing with the following relevant parameters: TR/TE = 3.0/1.5 ms, flip angle = 60°, field of view (FOV) of $(192\,\text{mm})^3$ with matrix size of 192^3 (voxel size = $1\,\text{mm}^3$). The continuous acquisition of a total of 60.480 projections were simulated. Based on previous publications [6], this corresponds to a simulated acquisition time of approximately 7 min. Respiratory and cardiac synchronization signal were provided by the numerical phantom and used to perform the double binning procedure described in Fig. 1b. The data was sorted into 4 respiratory states and 20 cardiac phases, leading to an average of 756 projections per reconstructed volume.

The reconstruction was carried out with the proposed method at an initial resolution of $4\,\text{mm}^3$ and at a second level of $2\,\text{mm}^3$ and with the original XD-GRASP approach at $2\,\text{mm}^3$ for comparison purposes. The NESTA algorithm [2] was used to solve the optimization problems in Eqs. (6) and (7). The parameter λ was fixed to 0.01 by visual inspection, so it is necessary to perform a complete validation study about this parameter in future works. A median filter of size 3^3 was applied to the final results to eliminate residual reconstructions artifacts. The equivalent acceleration factor (AF) was 6.08 for the low resolution level and 24.16 for the final one.

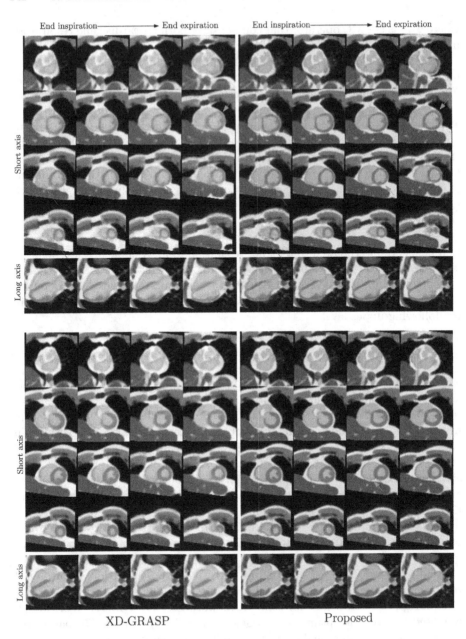

Fig. 3. Reconstructions of the XCAT phantom with XD-GRASP (left) and the proposed method with MC at diastole (top) and systole (bottom). Original volumes were reformatted to obtain four short axis slices covering the whole heart and one long axis slice. Data was binned in four respiratory states (from left to right). (Color figure online)

In order to validate the MC-XD approach on a real anatomy an isotropic 3D+t cardiac MR scan of a swine has also been used to obtain MC-XD MRI reconstruction by using the general scheme in Fig. 1 (without the multiresolution strategy). Due to the nature of these animals, respiratory motion is not appreciated in MRI, so a spatiotemporal deformation was synthetically generated to simulate different respiratory positions. Thus, a through-plane respiratory motion is modelled by a 2D gaussian function centred in the heart together with a XCAT respiratory signal in the temporal domain. Relevant imaging parameters include: voxel size = $1\,mm^3$, field of view = $183\,mm^3$, temporal resolution = 43 ms. The acquisition of a total number of 12.831 spokes was simulated and data sorted as with the phantom data, leading to an AF of 34.8.

3   Results and Discussion

In Fig. 3 the volumes reconstructed with XD-GRASP and the proposed method with MC are shown for the diastolic and systolic cardiac phases, for the four respiratory states in which the data was binned. A set of four short axis and one long axis slices were reformatted from the isotropic, unplanned volumes. In the images reconstructed with the proposed method, better contrast between blood pool and myocardium and sharped edges are recovered (green arrows), although these improvements are difficult to quantify. In fact, sharpness metrics such us that described in [9] produces similar values for images reconstructed with XD-GRASP and with the proposed method (49 and 47 in average, respectively), and it is not representative of the better image quality visually found in the reconstruction with the proposed method that has been highlighted in Fig. 3. However, high frequency artifacts can be appreciated in some areas in the results of the proposed method (red arrows). In these areas, the XD-GRASP reconstructions present strong blurring possibly due to residual *intrabin* motion than hinders the estimation of the cardio-respiratory motion. Similar artifacts have been previously reported for other MC related methods [16].

Figure 4 shows the obtained results for the swine MRI. XD-GRASP and MC reconstructions are presented for comparison. Better edge delineation, finer details and higher overall quality are appreciated in the case of images reconstructed with MC.

The reconstruction times for the synthetic data were 6.2 min for the initial low-resolution step, 7.1 min for the ME and 1.2 h for the final reconstruction. The same procedure directly applied to the final resolution level (not shown) took 23,6 min for the initial step, 10.85 min and 1.6 h for the MC reconstruction. Overall, the reconstruction time was 1.42 h for the multi-resolution scheme and 2.17 h for the other case, leading to a reduction of 34%.

SYSTOLE   DIASTOLE

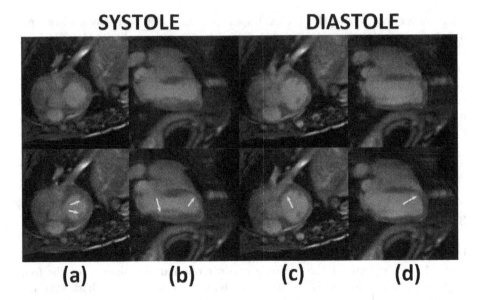

(a)   (b)   (c)   (d)

Fig. 4. Reconstructions of swine MRI (general scheme Fig. 1) for 60,480 acquired spokes (2,880 golden-angle-rotated interleaves with 21 spokes each, leading to a mean AF = 34.8 per reconstructed volume). Short axis views (a, c) and long axis views (b, d) of the heart for both systolic (a, b) and diastolic (c, d) phases. Initial CS reconstruction (XD-GRASP) is shown in top images; whereas the bottom images show the corresponding proposed MC-XD reconstruction. Yellow arrows indicate areas where the improvement in the recovered details with MC can be observed. (Color figure online)

4   Conclusion

This paper proposes an efficient extension of the XD MRI reconstruction. On one hand, a ME/MC approach based on a groupwise temporal registration is introduced in the reconstruction procedure, which allows to obtain a better edge definition in the obtained results. The obtained results have been compared with the XD-GRASP solution to support this affirmation.

On the other hand, a multi-resolution procedure has been designed to significantly reduce the computational cost of the MC-XD reconstruction process with similar image quality after reconstruction. The tests have shown a reduction of 34% in the overall reconstruction time for the proposed approach. Future works will focus on the validation of these results and the inclusion of solutions to avoid the presence of reconstruction artifacts, as it is already proposed in [17].

Acknowledgement. This work is partially supported by the Spanish Ministerio de Economía, Industria y Competitividad (MINECO) and by the Junta de Castilla y León through grants TEC201457428R and VA069U16, respectively.

References

1. Asif, M.S., Hamilton, L., Brummer, M., Romberg, J.: Motion-adaptive spatio-temporal regularization for accelerated dynamic MRI. Magn. Reson. Med. **70**(3), 800–812 (2013)
2. Becker, S., Bobin, J., Candes, E.J.: Nesta: a fast and accurate first-order method for sparse recovery. SIAM J. Imaging Sci. **4**(1), 1–39 (2011)
3. Chun, S.Y., Fessler, J.A.: A simple regularizer for b-spline nonrigid image registration that encourages local invertibility. IEEE J. Sel. Top. Sig. Process. **3**(1), 159–169 (2009)
4. Feng, L., et al.: Synchronized cardiac and respiratory sparsity for rapid free-breathing cardiac cine MRI. J. Cardiovasc. Magn. Reson. **16**(1), W26 (2014)
5. Feng, L., et al.: Xd-grasp: golden-angle radial MRI with reconstruction of extra motion-state dimensions using compressed sensing. Magn. Reson. Med. **75**(2), 775–788 (2016)
6. Feng, L., et al.: 5D whole-heart sparse MRI. Magn. Reson. Med. 1–13 (2017)
7. Jung, H., et al.: k-t focuss: a general compressed sensing framework for high resolution dynamic MRI. Magn. Reson. Med. **61**(1), 103–116 (2009)
8. Jung, H., Ye, J.C.: Motion estimated and compensated compressed sensing dynamic magnetic resonance imaging: what we can learn from video compression techniques. Int. J. Imaging Syst. Technol. **20**(2), 81–98 (2010)
9. Leclaire, A., Moisan, L.: No-reference image quality assessment and blind deblurring with sharpness metrics exploiting fourier phase information. J. Math. Imaging and Vis. **52**(1), 145–172 (2015). http://dx.doi.org/10.1007/s10851-015-0560-5
10. Piccini, D., Littmann, A., Nielles-Vallespin, S., Zenge, M.O.: Spiral phyllotaxis: the natural way to construct a 3D radial trajectory in MRI. Magn. Reson. Med. **66**(4), 1049–1056 (2011). http://dx.doi.org/10.1002/mrm.22898
11. Prieto, C., et al.: Reconstruction of undersampled dynamic images by modeling the motion of object elements. Magn. Reson. Med. **57**(5), 939–949 (2007)
12. Pruessmann, K.P., Weiger, M., Scheidegger, M.B., Boesiger, P.: Sense: sensitivity encoding for fast MRI. Magn. Reson. Med. **42**(5), 952–962 (1999)
13. Segars, W.P., Sturgeon, G., Mendonca, S., Grimes, J., Tsui, B.M.W.: 4d xcat phantom for multimodality imaging research. Med. Phys. **37**(9), 4902–4915 (2010)
14. Usman, M., et al.: Motion corrected compressed sensing for free-breathing dynamic cardiac MRI. Magn. Reson. Med. **70**(2), 504–516 (2013)
15. Royuela-del Val, J., et al.: Single breath hold whole heart cine MRI with iterative groupwise cardiac motion compensation and sparse regularization (kt-wise). In: Proceedings of the International Society for Magnetic Resonance in Medicine 23 (2015)
16. Royuela-del Val, J., et al.: Nonrigid groupwise registration for motion estimation and compensation in compressed sensing reconstruction of breath-hold cardiac cine mri. Magn. Reson. Med. **75**(4), 1525–1536 (2016)
17. Royuela-del Val, J., et al.: Jacobian weighted temporal total variation for motion compensated compressed sensing reconstruction of dynamic MRI. Magn. Reson. Med. **77**(3), 1208–1215 (2017)
18. Wissmann, L., et al.: Mrxcat: realistic numerical phantoms for cardiovascular magnetic resonance. J. Cardiovasc. Magn. Reson. **16**(1), 63 (2014)

First International Stroke Workshop on Imaging and Treatment Challenges, SWITCH 2017

Automated Ventricular System Segmentation in CT Images of Deformed Brains Due to Ischemic and Subarachnoid Hemorrhagic Stroke

E. Ferdian[1,2,3(✉)] , A.M. Boers[1,2,4] , L.F. Beenen[2] ,
B.M. Cornelissen[1,2,4] , I.G. Jansen[2] , K.M. Treurniet[2] ,
J. Borst[2] , C.B. Majoie[2] , and H.A. Marquering[1,2]

[1] Department of Biomedical Engineering and Physics, Academic Medical Center,
Meibergdreef 15, Amsterdam, The Netherlands
edwardferdian03@gmail.com
[2] Department of Radiology, Academic Medical Center,
Meibergdreef 15, Amsterdam, The Netherlands
[3] Department of Medical Informatics, Academic Medical Center,
Meibergdreef 15, Amsterdam, The Netherlands
[4] Department of Robotics and Mechatronics, University of Twente,
Hallenweg 15, Enschede, The Netherlands

Abstract. Accurate ventricle segmentation is important for reliable automated infarct localization, detection of early ischemic changes, and localization of hemorrhages. The purpose of this study was to develop a robust and accurate ventricle segmentation method in image data of ischemic and hemorrhagic stroke patients. Early follow-up non-contrast CT image data of 35 patients with a clinical diagnosis of ischemic stroke or subarachnoid hemorrhage were collected. We proposed a ventricle segmentation method based on a combination of active contours and an atlas-based segmentation. Ground truth was obtained by manual delineation of the ventricles by 4 observers with corrections by 2 experienced radiologists. Accuracy of the automated method was evaluated by calculation of the intraclass correlation coefficients, Dice coefficients, and by Bland-Altman analysis. The intraclass correlation coefficient for the automated method compared with the reference standard was excellent (0.93). The Dice coefficients was 0.79 [IQR: 0.72–0.84]. Bland-Altman analysis showed a mean difference of 2 mL between the automatic and manual measurements, with broad limits of agreement ranging from −18 to 15 mL. The automated ventricle segmentation showed an excellent correlation and high accuracy compared to the manual reference measurement. This approach is suitable for reliable ventricle segmentation even in stroke patients with a severely deformed brain.

Keywords: Ventricular system · Segmentation · Deformed brain · CT · Stroke · Subarachnoid hemorrhage

© Springer International Publishing AG 2017
M.J. Cardoso et al. (Eds.): CMMI/RAMBO/SWITCH 2017, LNCS 10555, pp. 149–157, 2017.
DOI: 10.1007/978-3-319-67564-0_15

1 Introduction

Stroke is the leading cause of disability and second leading cause of death worldwide [1]. Diagnosis and treatment decisions of patients with ischemic and hemorrhagic stroke depend heavily on radiological imaging. Recently, various automated methods of CT image analysis of stroke patients have been introduced: infarct core quantification [2], hemorrhage quantification [3], and ASPECTS scoring [4]. In these methods, accurate ventricle segmentation plays a key role in correctly locating and quantifying these lesions.

Several methods have been proposed for segmenting the ventricles either in healthy or slightly deformed brains. These methods were based on techniques such as region growing [5, 6], cognition network [7], low-level segmentation combined with high-level template matching [8], and active model-based segmentation [9–11]. In stroke patients, severe deformation of the brain is quite common. However, this deformation issue is not normally addressed in existing literatures. In general, ventricle segmentation for stroke patients shared a common trait, such as difficulty in distinguishing infarct regions from the ventricles due to similar intensity and also the stroke regions are often located adjacent to the ventricle. For example, in ischemic stroke patients, the density of infarct regions can be in the proximity of that of cerebrospinal fluid (CSF) within the ventricles. Moreover, in other cases such as hemorrhagic stroke, blood often leaks inside the ventricles, yielding problems with existing segmentation methods.

Up to now, only several ventricle segmentation methods that are dedicated for stroke patients have been proposed [10, 12, 13]. These studies, however, focused on either ischemic or hemorrhagic stroke patients, but not both. We tried to take an approach from the perspective of brain deformation due to stroke.

The aim of our study was to design a robust automated ventricular segmentation method for CT images suitable for patients with severe brain deformation due to ischemic or subarachnoid hemorrhagic stroke to aid subsequent image analyses, such as infarct quantification and subarachnoid hemorrhage detection tools.

2 Materials and Methods

2.1 Patient Selection

Early follow-up whole-brain non-contrast CT (NCCT) image data of 50 patients with a clinical diagnosis of ischemic stroke or subarachnoid hemorrhage (SAH) were collected. Brain image data with 5 mm slice thickness were used, resulting in volumes with 24–51 slices. We retrieved 1-week follow-up NCCT image data of ischemic stroke patients from the MR CLEAN database [14], while baseline NCCT image data of SAH patients were retrieved from the local data base from our institute. From our initial image database of 50 patients, patients with hemicraniectomy (n = 4) and incomplete image data (n = 11) were excluded. The image data were anonymized before analyses.

2.2 Method Overview

The proposed ventricle segmentation approach is based on localized region-based active contours [15]. Since active contours require a good initial estimation, we divided our method into two stages: (1) initial contour estimation using atlas-based ventricle segmentation and (2) active contours based ventricle segmentation.

First stage: Initial contour estimation. In the first stage, we performed an atlas-based segmentation on skull-stripped brain images. The skull-stripping algorithm is performed using a thresholding operation [3] to exclude the skull and non-brain tissues from the subject image. We considered regions >100 HU as the skull and excluded them from the brain image. Registrations were performed using open source software Elastix (version 4.3; http://elastix.isi.uu.nl) [16, 17] with mutual information set as similarity measure. Rigid, affine, and B-splined (grid spacing: 15 mm) transformations were applied sequentially. Subsequently, we applied the transformation parameter from the registered image to the ventricle atlas. For this purpose, we used an in-house-developed ventricle atlas that contains labels of the two lateral ventricles, third ventricle, fourth ventricle, and nonventricular CSF regions. The atlas-based segmentation resulted in masks of the ventricles of the patient image (See Fig. 1).

Subsequently in the masked areas, CSF and hemorrhage within the ventricles were segmented using density-based thresholding. All voxels within the masked image with a density of 0–16HU and 55–90HU were labeled as CSF and intraventricular blood respectively. Voxels with a density between 16 and 55 HU were considered as normal brain tissue.

The result of the procedure described above included false positives, which consist of adjacent infarct regions, adjacent hemorrhagic regions, and non-ventricular CSF regions, which mostly occur around the segmentation of lateral ventricles. To detect false positive regions, in every axial slice of the lateral ventricles, a connected component analysis was performed, subsequently followed by region growing operation on each of the components. The region growing was performed to include neighboring pixels with density slightly range slightly higher than the CSF segmentation [0–19 HU] to ensure connectivity to nonventricular CSF regions. When the result of region growing overlaps more than 75% with the original segmentation, the seed component is considered as a true positive. On the other hand, when the result spread towards previously unsegmented region, the component is removed from the original segmentation (See Fig. 2).

Second Stage: Active contours based ventricle segmentation. Localized region-based active contours was used in the refinement stage [15, 18]. Uniform energy modeling was used as internal energy measure. The foreground (CSF/ventricle) and background (white matter, gray matter) are modeled as constant intensity values represented by their means. Because of the large differences between in-plane resolution and slice thickness, active contours was applied in 2D axial slices rather than in a 3D volume, with the following parameters: radius of local area (rad = 10), coefficient curvature regularization term ($\alpha = 0.001$), smoothness ($\varepsilon = 10$), number of iterations (n = 500). This 2D approach also allowed the active contours to filter out small noise regions.

We first performed active contours on the main slice of the lateral ventricles. We defined the main slice as the axial slice that contains the largest two-dimensional (2D) connected component from the initial estimation. For the main slice, the initial segmentation from the previous stage is used as the initial contour. The segmentation result from the main slice is then used to calculate patient-specific CSF threshold. This segmentation result is propagated to its adjacent inferior and superior slices to be used as an input for the next initial contour.

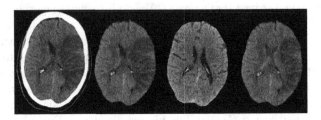

Fig. 1. Examples of atlas-based segmentation on a skull-stripped image (First column shows the original brain image with skull, second column shows the brain image without skull (regions >100 HU excluded), third column shows the registered image, fourth column shows atlas-based segmentation on the skull-stripped image).

Subsequently, the third, fourth, and the remainder of lateral ventricles slices were segmented using active contours in a propagative manner. This order was chosen due to the interconnectedness of the ventricle regions. To compensate to the large distance between slices, initial contours were obtained by combining the estimation from the first stage and the projection from the segmentation from the previous slice, masked with the patient-specific CSF threshold.

Finally, intraventricular calcification regions were identified to be included as ventricles in the segmentation. In slices that contain the posterior and inferior horns (axial slices between the roof of the 3rd and roof of the 4th ventricle); dilation morphological operation with a structuring element of 5×5 mm was applied to include calcifications.

2.3   Accuracy

Ventricles in 35 CT images (17 ischemic stroke and 18 SAH patient images) were manually delineated by trained observers and when necessary corrected by experienced radiologists (L.F.B and C.B.M, both with >10 years of experience). The manually delineated ventricles were used as reference standard to evaluate the accuracy of our method.

The accuracy was measured by calculating the Intraclass Correlation Coefficient (ICC) and performing Bland-Altman analysis. Furthermore, the Dice similarity coefficient (DSC) between the automated and manual segmentation was determined to calculate the overlap.

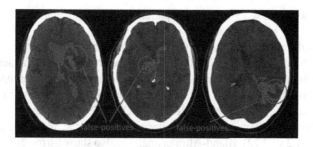

Fig. 2. Illustration of false-positives regions that were detected by region-growing algorithm. The component which was used as the seed is labelled as a potential leak and excluded from the refinement process

3   Results

The automated segmentation was successfully performed on all 35 NCCT images (17 ischemic stroke and 18 SAH patients) without any manual intervention or adjustment. The median ventricle volume was 33.2 mL [IQR: 23.7–43.2] and 28.1 mL [IQR: 25.5–45.9], according to the automated and manual delineations, respectively. The ventricle segmentation took 10–20 min per patient to complete on a Core i7, 2.67 GHz PC with 6 GB RAM. This execution time is without the time to perform the atlas-based

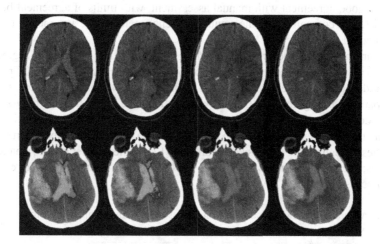

Fig. 3. Examples of segmented ventricles (1st column represents the original atlas-based segmentations with false-positive regions. The 2nd column represents the segmentations after removal of the false-positive regions. The 3rd column represents the final segmentations. The last column represents the delineations by experts, which was used as a reference standard). On the first and second column cyan represents the lateral ventricles, green and red represent non-ventricular CSF regions. On the third and fourth column red represents the final segmentation. The first and second row show ischemic and subarachnoid hemorrhagic stroke patient images, respectively. (Color figure online)

segmentation, which took 15–30 min per patient. Some segmentation results are shown in Fig. 3.

The ICC of the automatic and manual ventricle volume measurement was excellent: 0.93 (95%CI 0.88–0.96; p < 0.001). Bland-Altman analysis indicated a mean difference in ventricle volume of 2 mL between the automatic and manual measurements, with limits of agreement ranging from −18 to 15 mL. The Dice coefficient of the manual and automatic measurements had a median of 0.79 [IQR: 0.72–0.84]. Overall, the accuracy for segmentations in ischemic stroke is higher compared to the SAH patients (ICC: 0.97 vs 0.88, DSC: 0.82 vs 0.72). Bland-Altman analysis also show narrower limits of agreement in the ischemic stroke segmentation compared to the SAH (−10 to 9.6 mL as opposed to −24 to 17 mL). See Table 1.

Our method successfully distinguished between CSF and infarcts or hemorrhages. However, some minor leakages were still observed in 5 (14.3%) of the segmentations, for example into non-ventricular CSF regions, infarcts, and hemorrhages. Additionally, in some cases the proposed method did not recognize narrow or small regions such as the cerebral aqueduct between the third and fourth ventricle.

4   Discussion

We introduced an automated ventricle segmentation method in NCCT images of patients with ischemic stroke or SAH with a severely deformed brain. The segmentation method is fully automated and applicable to severely deformed brain. Evaluation with 35 patients showed a good agreement with manual assessment, with limits of agreement between −18 and 15 mL compared with the manual reference method. The accuracy of the automated method was high.

To our knowledge, the presented method is the first that is robust in segmenting ventricles in severely deformed brains for both ischemic stroke and SAH patients. Compared to previous methods [10, 12, 13], the accuracy of our method for ischemic stroke patients is slightly lower. However, it should be noted that we only selected severely deformed ventricles in our study. In addition, the presented method works well in a wide range of ventricle size from our sample data. Previous studies reported some difficulties in segmenting small sized ventricles [12], while in other studies smaller size ventricles, such as the fourth ventricle [7, 9, 11] and third ventricle [5] were excluded in the process.

Table 1. Accuracy of manual ventricle volume measurement and comparison of the manual and automated segmentation.

Segmentation	Intraclass correlation (95% CI)	Dice coefficient (median and IQR)	Bland-Altman limits of agreement (mL)	# samples
Automated vs manual	0.93 (0.88–0.96)	0.79 [IQR: 0.72–0.84]	−18–15	35
Automated vs manual (ischemic)	0.97 (0.93–0.99)	0.82 [IQR: 0.78–0.86]	−10–9.6	17
Automated vs manual (SAH)	0.88 (0.76–0.95)	0.72 [IQR: 0.64–0.77]	−24–17	18

Recent study from Qian et al. [13] showed an impressive result in segmenting ventricle and distinguishing stroke regions. However, we find that the method relies on symmetry of the brain which is not often the case for severely deformed brain. Moreover, we tried to generalize our method to cover different cases of stroke and not specific to ischemic stroke.

We used atlas based segmentation for our initial contours by performing non-linear registration on skull-stripped brain images. We found this approach suitable for our cases with deformed brain. Other approaches, such as the above mentioned symmetric based approach is not suitable for our dataset. In terms of active contours segmentation, we used a propagated 2D approach instead of 3D approach in order to detect leaking as early as possible. By putting a size threshold on the contours, the extent of leakage is minimized. The novelty of our method lies in the removal of false-positives using region-growing algorithm. We took advantage of the leaking characteristics of region growing to detect false-positive segmentations.

In our study, we have chosen to develop a method that allows the segmentation of severely deformed ventricles for both ischemic stroke as well as subarachnoid hemorrhage patients. Alternatively, it could also be possible to combine two different segmentation techniques that are optimized for either ischemic stroke or subarachnoid hemorrhages and select the optimal result retrospectively. However, it was beyond the scope of this study to explore this strategy.

There are a few limitations in our method. Our method is computationally demanding. Even though the localized region-based active contours has shorter computation time compared to the global variant [15], our implementation took around 20–30 min per patient. A limitation is that we evaluated the accuracy on the same image data set as was used for its development. This may, therefore, overestimate its accuracy. Because of the limited number of severely deformed ventricles, we used the same dataset for both training and evaluation purposes.

Using our method, the accuracy of the segmentation in SAH patients was somewhat lower compared to ischemic stroke patients. In SAH patients, there is commonly a large amount of blood within or adjacent to the ventricle, especially around the posterior and inferior horns. The ventricle segmentation is the most difficult for these patients because of the indistinct boundary between intra-and-extra ventricular hemorrhages.

This automated approach enables a reproducible and observer-independent analysis. Our method offers the following improvements compared to previously presented methods: complete segmentation of all ventricles (lateral, third, and fourth ventricles), accurate in patients with subarachnoid hemorrhages, and a control to prevent excessive segmentation leakage to infarct and non-ventricular CSF regions.

There is still some room for improvement. Future work may address improvement of the initial contour estimation, reduction of computation time of the active contours, and improvement in the detection of intra vs. extra-ventricular hemorrhages.

We have presented a robust automatic method for ventricle segmentation in CT images of ischemic stroke and SAH patients with severely deformed brains. The segmentation accuracy is sufficient to assist additional automated methods that require ventricle segmentation such as the detection of infarcts and subarachnoid hemorrhages.

References

1. Towfighi, A., Saver, J.L.: Stroke declines from third to fourth leading cause of death in the United States: historical perspective and challenges ahead. Stroke **42**, 2351–2355 (2011). doi: 10.1161/STROKEAHA.111.621904
2. Boers, A.M., Marquering, H.A., Jochem, J.J., et al.: Automated cerebral infarct volume measurement in follow-up noncontrast CT scans of patients with acute ischemic stroke. Am. J Neuroradiol. **34**, 1522–1527 (2013). doi:10.3174/ajnr.A3463
3. Boers, A.M., Zijlstra, I.A., Gathier, C.S., et al.: Automatic quantification of subarachnoid hemorrhage on noncontrast CT. Am. J. Neuroradiol. **35**, 2279–2286 (2014). doi:10.3174/ajnr.A4042
4. Stoel, B.C., Marquering, H.A., Staring, M., et al.: Automated brain CT densitometry of early ischemic changes in acute stroke. AJNR Am. J. Neuroradiol. (2013). doi:10.1117/1.JMI. 2.1.014004
5. Schnack, H.G., Hulshoff Pol, H.E., Baaré, W.F.C., et al.: Automatic segmentation of the ventricular system from MR images of the human brain. Neuroimage **14**, 95–104 (2001). doi: 10.1006/nimg.2001.080
6. Xia, Y., Hu, Q., Aziz, A., Nowinski, W.L.: A knowledge-driven algorithm for a rapid and automatic extraction of the human cerebral ventricular system from MR neuroimages. Neuroimage **21**, 269–282 (2004). doi:10.1016/j.neuroimage.2003.09.029
7. Schönmeyer, R., Prvulovic, D., Rotarska-Jagiela, A., et al.: Automated segmentation of lateral ventricles from human and primate magnetic resonance images using cognition network technology. Magn. Reson. Imaging **24**, 1377–1387 (2006). doi:10.1016/j.mri.2006.08.013
8. Chen, W., Smith, R., Ji, S.-Y., et al.: Automated ventricular systems segmentation in brain CT images by combining low-level segmentation and high-level template matching. BMC Med. Inform. Decis. Mak. **9**, S4 (2009). doi:10.1186/1472-6947-9-S1-S4
9. Fan, Y., Jiang, T., Evans, D.J.: Volumetric segmentation of brain images using parallel genetic algorithms. IEEE Trans. Med. Imaging **21**, 904–909 (2002). doi:10.1109/TMI.2002.803126
10. Liu, J., Huang, S., Ihar, V., et al.: Automatic model-guided segmentation of the human brain ventricular system from CT images. Acad. Radiol. **17**, 718–726 (2010). doi:10.1016/j.acra. 2010.02.013
11. Etyngier, P., Ségonne, F., Keriven, R.: Active-contour-based image segmentation using machine learning techniques. In: Ayache, N., Ourselin, S., Maeder, A. (eds.) MICCAI 2007. LNCS, vol. 4791, pp. 891–899. Springer, Heidelberg (2007). doi:10.1007/978-3-540-75757-3_108
12. Poh, L.E., Gupta, V., Johnson, A., et al.: Automatic segmentation of ventricular cerebrospinal fluid from ischemic stroke CT images. Neuroinformatics **10**, 159–172 (2012). doi:10.1007/s12021-011-9135-9
13. Qian, X., Lin, Y., Zhao, Y., et al.: Objective ventricle segmentation in brain CT with ischemic stroke based on anatomical knowledge. Biomed. Res. Int. **2017**, 1–11 (2017). doi: 10.1155/2017/8690892
14. Berkhemer, O., Fransen, P., Beumer, D., et al.: A randomized trial of intraarterial treatment for acute ischemic stroke. New. Engl. J. Med. **372**, 11–20 (2014). doi:10.1056/NEJMoa1411587
15. Lankton, S., Tannenbaum, A.: Localizing region-based active contours. IEEE Trans. Image Process. **17**, 2029–2039 (2008). doi:10.1109/TIP.2008.2004611
16. Klein, S., Staring, M., Murphy, K., et al.: Elastix: a toolbox for intensity-based medical image registration. IEEE Trans. Med. Imaging **29**, 196–205 (2010)

17. Shamonin, D.P., Bron, E.E., Lelieveldt, B.P.F., et al.: Fast parallel image registration on CPU and GPU for diagnostic classification of Alzheimer's disease. Front. Neuroinform. **7**, 50 (2013)
18. Pang, J.: Localized Active Contour (2014). http://uk.mathworks.com/matlabcentral/fileexchange/44906-localized-active-contour

Towards Automatic Collateral Circulation Score Evaluation in Ischemic Stroke Using Image Decompositions and Support Vector Machines

Yiming Xiao[1,2(✉)], Ali Alamer[3], Vladimir Fonov[4], Benjamin W.Y. Lo[5], Donatella Tampieri[3,5], D. Louis Collins[4], Hassan Rivaz[1,2], and Marta Kersten-Oertel[1,6]

[1] PERFORM Centre, Concordia University, Montreal, Canada
yiming.xiao@concordia.ca
[2] Department of Electrical and Computer Engineering, Concordia University, Montreal, Canada
[3] Diagnostic and Interventional Neuroradiology, Montreal Neurological Hospital, Montreal, Canada
[4] McConnell Brain Imaging Centre, Montreal Neurological Institute, Montreal, Canada
[5] Department of Neurology and Neurosurgery, Montreal Neurological Hospital, Montreal, Canada
[6] Department of Computer Science and Software Engineering, Concordia University, Montreal, Canada

Abstract. Stroke is the second leading cause of disability worldwide. Thrombectomy has been shown to offer fast and efficient reperfusion with high recanalization rates and thus improved patient outcomes. One of the most important indicators to identify patients amenable to thrombectomy is evidence of good collateral circulation. Currently, methods for evaluating collateral circulation are generally limited to visual inspection with potentially high inter- and intra-rater variability. In this work, we present an automatic technique to evaluate collateral circulation. This is achieved via low-rank decomposition of the target subject's 4D CT angiography, and using principal component analysis (PCA) and support vector machines (SVMs) to automatically generate a collateral circulation score. With the proposed automatic score evaluation technique, we have achieved an overall scoring accuracy of 82.2% to identify patients with poor, intermediate, and good/normal collateral circulation.

Keywords: CTA · Collateral score · Stroke · Machine learning

1 Introduction

According to the World Heart Federation, each year over 15 million people suffer from brain stroke, with 6 million dying as a result, and 5 million becoming permanently disabled[1]. The two main types of stroke are: (1) hemorrhagic, due to bleeding, and (2) ischemic, due to a lack of blood flow. In this paper, we focus on ischemic stroke, which

---

[1] http://www.world-heart-federation.org/cardiovascular-health/stroke/.

© Springer International Publishing AG 2017
M.J. Cardoso et al. (Eds.): CMMI/RAMBO/SWITCH 2017, LNCS 10555, pp. 158–167, 2017.
DOI: 10.1007/978-3-319-67564-0_16

accounts for approximately 87% of all stroke cases. In ischemic stroke, where poor blood flow to the brain causes neuronal cell death, the goal of treatment is to restore blood flow to preserve tissue in the ischemic penumbra, where blood flow is decreased but sufficient enough to stave off infarction (i.e. cell death).

It has been shown that recanalization, i.e. restoring blood flow, is the most important modifiable prognostic predictor for a favorable outcome in ischemic stroke [1]. Timely restoration of regional blood flow can help salvage threatened tissue, reducing cell death, and ultimately minimizing patient disabilities. Thrombectomy, where a long catheter with a mechanical device attached to the tip, is used to remove a clot, has been effective for treatment for ischemic stroke. However, the inherent risks associated with thrombectomy must be considered, and only patients with certain indications, including a large penumbra, small infarct, and sufficient collateral circulation should undergo such interventions. Collateral circulation (i.e., collaterals) is defined as a supplementary vascular network that is dynamically recruited when there is an arterial occlusion (e.g. a clot) and has been shown to be one of the most important factors in determining treatment strategies [2, 3].

Currently, collaterals are typically evaluated on Computed Tomography Angiography (CTA) or Magnetic Resonance Angiography (MRA), however, there is no consensus on which imaging modality should be used [4]. For assessment on CTA, a collateral score is based on visual inspection of the images by a radiologist and can be graded using scoring systems, such as the Alberta Stroke Program Early CT Score (ASPECTS) [5]. However, visual inspection is often subject to inter- and intra-rater inconsistency and can be time-consuming. To the best our knowledge, no automatic collateral score evaluation methods have been reported previously in the literature.

In this paper, we present an automatic technique for estimating the collateral score in dynamic 4D CTA images. First, blood vessel patterns are extracted using low-rank image decompositions, and then collateral scores are assigned using support vector machines (SVMs) based on eigen blood vessel patterns from principal component analysis (PCA). To demonstrate the performance of SVMs for the task, we compared the results against classification using k-nearest neighbors (kNN) and random forests.

2 Materials and Methods

2.1 Subjects and Scanning Protocols

For this study, we included 29 patients who had suffered a stroke and 8 healthy subjects. For all subjects (age = 65 ± 15 yo), isotropic computed tomography (CT) imaging was acquired on Toshiba's Aquilion ONE 320-row detector 640-slice cone beam CT (Toshiba medical systems, Tokyo, Japan). The time between symptoms onset and scanning varies, but for most it is within 24 h. The routine stroke protocol uses a series of intermittent volume scans over a period of 60 s with a scanning speed of 0.75 s/rotation. This protocol provides whole brain perfusion and whole brain dynamic vascular analysis in one examination. A total of 18 volumes are acquired, where a series of low-dose scans are performed: first for every two seconds during the arterial phase, and then spaced out to every 5 s to capture the slower venous phase of the contrast bolus. Isovue-370

(Iopamidol) is used as non-ionic and low osmolar contrast medium (Iodine content, 370 mg/ml).

2.2 Collateral Circulation Scoring for Patients

The collateral circulations of the 29 patients were scored by two radiologists as being *good*, *intermediate* or *poor* using the Alberta Stroke Program Early CT score (ASPECTS) [5]. The scoring criteria are as follows: a score of *good* is given for 100% collateral supply of the occluded middle cerebral artery (MCA) territory; *intermediate* score is given when collateral supply fills more than 50% but less then 100% of the occluded MCA territory; a *poor* score indicates collateral supply that fills less then 50% but more than 0% of the occluded MCA territory (Fig. 1). Among the patients, we had 9 *good*, 14 *intermediate*, and 6 *poor* subjects.

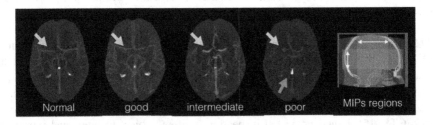

Fig. 1. Examples of axial maximum intensity projections (MIPs) for different collateral circulation scores. The middle cerebral artery (MCA) is annotated with yellow arrows, and the blue arrow points to calcification at the pituitary gland. The MCA territory is to the lateral region of the MCAs. The blue and green regions are the projection regions in the coronal and axial directions that will be used for automatic collateral score computation. (Color figure online)

2.3 Image Processing

Each subject's 18 CTAs were first rigidly co-registered together, and then spatially normalized to a population-averaged CTA template created using the first CTA of the series (with the least blood vessel contrast) with nonlinear registration. The registrations help ensure all brains were in the same space for analysis, and were completed with the freely available Advanced Normalization Tools (ANTs) (stnava.github.io/ANTs). The template was created from 11 healthy subjects that had undergone the same dynamic 4D-CTA imaging protocol. Individual averaged CTAs were deformed and averaged together through an unbiased group-wise registration scheme as described in [6]. The resulting template, with a resolution of $1 \times 1 \times 1$ mm^3, is shown in Fig. 2. A brain mask was extracted from the template using the active contour segmentation tool in ITK-SNAP (www.itksnap.org) and used for the analysis of individual brain volumes.

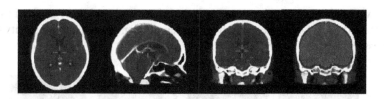

Fig. 2. Population-averaged non-linear template (From left to right: axial, sagittal and coronal views). The brain mask is shown overlaid on the coronal view in the rightmost image.

2.4 Blood Vessel Extraction

The evaluation of collateral circulation is largely determined by the flow of contrast agent in the blood vessels over time. However, within the CTA images, other brain anatomy, such as the ventricles and grey matter are still visible. To remove non-vessel structures that exhibit inter-subject variability and can affect the PCA results intended only for blood vessels, we employed low-rank decomposition. Previously, low-rank decomposition has been used to separate foreground and background in a scene from video footages [7]. In this case, each image in the series can be modeled as the summation of the low-rank components that contain consistent anatomical structures across time, and a sparsity term that describes the intensity changes in the blood vessels. For a subject k, the 4D CTAs are stored in a matrix $D = \left[I_k^1, .., I_k^i, ..., I_k^{18}\right]$, where I_k^i is the ith CTA image that is converted to a column vector from the time series. The low-rank representation of D is defined as:

$$\left\{\widehat{L}, \widehat{S}\right\} = argmin_{L,S}\left(rank(L) + \gamma\|S\|_0\right) \ subject \ to \ D = L + S \qquad (1)$$

where $\|S\|_0$ is the counting norm of the sparsity component S, rank(L) is the matrix rank of the low-rank component L, and γ is a positive scalar. To make the optimization tractable, the problem is then transformed as:

$$\left\{\widehat{L}, \widehat{S}\right\} = argmin_{L,S}\left(\|L\|_* + \rho\|S\|_1\right) \ subject \ to \ D = L + S \qquad (2)$$

where $\|L\|_*$ is the nuclear norm of L, $\|S\|_1$ is the L1-norm of S, and ρ is a positive scalar that controls the approximated rank of matrix L. There have been many methods to solve this optimization problem. For our application, we employed the augmented Lagrange multiplier method [8] to recover the low-rank and sparsity components. As a result, each image I_k^i is represented as $I_k^i = l_k^i + s_k^i$, where l_k^i and s_k^i are the low-rank and sparse representation of I_k^i. For our application, to reduce image noise and inter-subject anatomical variability (i.e., blood vessels), the CTA images were first blurred by a Gaussian kernel of $\sigma = 3\,mm$ (the thickness of main arteries), and then processed with low-rank decomposition. All sparse representations for each subject's CTA series were averaged. Lastly, the median value projection in the axial direction and mean value projection in the coronal direction were obtained using the projection regions in Fig. 1. They were then used to extract eigen vessel patterns. Examples of the projections are shown in Fig. 3. Note that on the left hemisphere, as the blood circulation worsens, the intensity of the blood vessels becomes lower.

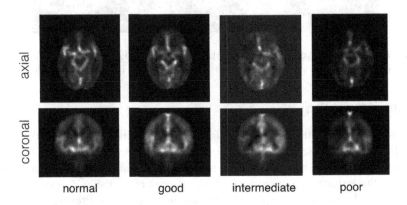

Fig. 3. Examples of 2D projection images (axial view: median value in axial direction, coronal view: mean value in coronal direction) for the typical normal, good, intermediate and poor collateral circulation.

2.5   Eigen Vessel Patterns and Score Assignment

Principal component analysis (PCA) has been commonly used for object recognition [9] through the generation of eigen image basis. From the training set composed of selected vectorized image features $X = [X_1, X_2, \ldots, X_m] \subset \mathfrak{R}^{n \times m}$, the covariance matrix C can be decomposed into $C = U \Lambda U^T$, with Λ being the diagonal matrix containing the eigenvalues $\{\lambda_a\}_{a=1 \ldots N}$ and U being the orthonormal matrix that has the corresponding principal components (or eigen vessel patterns) $\{\emptyset_a\}_{a=1 \ldots N}$. When a new image ψ is presented, it can be represented as $\psi = \overline{X} + \sum_{a=1}^{N} w_a \phi_a$, where the reconstruction coefficient can be found via $w_a = \phi_a^T (\psi - \overline{X})$ and $\overline{X} = \frac{1}{m} \sum_{j}^{m} X_j$. As we have images from coronal and axial direction projections for subject K, two sets of reconstruction coefficients $w_{coronal}^k$ and w_{axial}^k were concatenated as $w^k = [w_{coronal}^k, w_{axial}^k]$ to feed into multi-class SVMs with the radial basis function (RBF) kernel and one-vs-all scheme [10] to assign each subject with a collateral score. For a binary SVM classifier, the decision function is defined as $f(w) = \sum y_i \alpha_i K(w, w_i) + b$, where the kernel $K(x_i, x_j) = \exp\left(\beta \|x_i - x_j\|^2\right)$ is the radial basis function, w_i is the support vector, y_i is the binary class label, and α_i and b are the coefficients and bias term to be trained. In the one-vs-all type scheme, a binary SVM is trained for each class to separate the examples in the target class (positive labeled) from the remaining ones (negative labeled). For a new subject to be classified, the axial and coronal projection images are first projected to the eigen vessel patterns obtained from the training data, and the associated feature vector w is produced by concatenating the reconstruction coefficients. Lastly, the feature vector w is classified with the associated classifier that has the highest score computed from all classifiers.

2.6 Training and Validation

As there is almost no visual difference between the 4D CTAs of normal controls and patients with collateral scores of good, we combined them as one group for training and classification. Therefore, we categorized all the subjects into three classes: good/normal, intermediate, and poor. As there are much fewer subjects with poor collateral circulation and it is desirable to have a balanced dataset for training, we generated 8 more new subjects by nonlinearly registering these cases to normal controls with the least anatomical similarity to them. We used CTA images that contain general brain anatomy and clear vasculature for registration. This way, we ensure that the synthesized anatomy is distinct from both the original image and the image to be registered to. To further enrich the training set, we also included the left-and-right mirrored versions of the subjects since most often a stroke occurs unilaterally, and the equal chance of having a stroke on the left or right hemisphere should be represented. Finally, we employed a leave-one-out scheme to validate our computer-assisted scoring system. However, as the dataset contains both the original and mirrored images, we only validated the classification results for 45 original images in order to avoid repeated classification. More specifically, for each target subject to receive a score, the subject's images (both original and mirrored versions) will be excluded from the training set. This leaves 88 subjects to generate the eigen vessel patterns and train the classifier at each round of validation. To assess the performance of the SVMs for collateral scoring, with the same image features, we compared the classification results using SVMs against those using k-nearest neighbors (kNN) and random forests. More specifically, through cross-validation, in terms of overall scoring accuracy, we found that for kNN, the optimal number of neighbors is 7, and for random forests, 150 trees offer the best results.

3 Results

3.1 Low-Rank Image Decomposition

A demonstration of low-rank decomposition is shown in Fig. 4 for two different subjects. Compared with the original image, the pattern of blood vessels is captured in the sparsity component while the other brain anatomy and calcification in the falx (Subject 1) have been removed. As for Subject 2 with poor collateral circulation, the absence of bright blood vessels on the right hemisphere can be observed in the sparsity component.

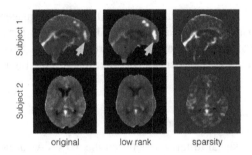

Fig. 4. Demonstration of low-rank decomposition using two subjects (different from those in Fig. 3). The yellow arrows point to the calcifications, and the vasculatures are shown as bright signals in the sparsity images. (Color figure online)

3.2 Eigen Vessel Patterns

The first 5 most significant principal components (or eigen vessel patterns) ranked by the eigenvalues for the two projections are shown in Fig. 5. Note that the asymmetric eigen vessel patterns in Fig. 5 are the results of unilateral collateral clots.

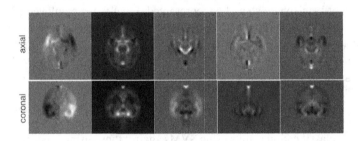

Fig. 5. Eigen blood vessel patterns of axial and coronal projection images.

3.3 Automatic Collateral Circulation Scoring Results

The score assignment accuracy for each class and in total are show in Table 1 for the SVMs, random forests, and k-nearest neighbors. In general, the SVMs achieved higher scoring accuracy than the other two methods. To better understand the classification results with SVMs, the related confusion matrix is shown in Table 2.

4   Discussion and Future Work

We used low-rank decomposition to extract vasculatures from the 4D CTA for three reasons. First, compared with simple subtraction of pre- and post-contrast CTAs, low-rank decomposition does not increase the image noise level. Second, the method can remove or mitigate unwanted image features, such as hyperintense signals from the calcifications in the pituitary gland, ventricles or the falx. Lastly, the method preserves the relative image intensity changes due to blood circulation while removing other anatomical features. We employed 2D projection images for the classification task. Compared with directly using 3D volumes, which achieved overall scoring accuracy of 73.3%, 46.7% and 46.7% for SVMs, random forests, and kNN techniques, respectively, the 2D approach requires less computational burden, and performs better likely due to further reduction of blood vessel anatomical variability from projection. Here, the projection methods are chosen with the consideration of the blood flow direction (from bottom to top of the brain). When a clot occurs, the superior side of the MCA territory will appear dark, and the more severe the case is, the less blood reaches the region. As a result, the coronal mean projection captures the blood supply perpendicular to the flow direction while the axial median projection measures the property along flow direction. Compared with the selected projection methods, the conventional MIPs did not perform as well (71.1%, 55.6%, and 57.8% overall classification accuracy for SVMs, kNN, and random forests).

Table 1. Evaluation of collateral circulation score classification accuracy

	Normal/Good	Intermediate	Poor	All
SVMs	82.4%	64.3%	100%	82.2%
Random forest	64.7%	42.9%	85.7%	64.4%
kNN	41.2%	42.9%	85.7%	55.6%

Table 2. Confusion matrix for collateral score classification results using SVMs.

Prediction	True class		
	Normal/Good	Intermediate	Poor
Normal/Good	14	2	0
Intermediate	2	9	0
Poor	1	3	14

For this work, we only had a small cohort of subjects available, yet the cerebral vasculature has much higher variability than other anatomical structures in the brain. Therefore, we blurred the CTA images using a Gaussian kernel with a kernel size of 3 mm, which is the diameter of the main cerebral arteries, to reduce the variability of the smaller vessels. For training, we synthesized new subjects with poor collateral circulation due to a highly imbalanced dataset. Since nonlinear registration will significantly alter anatomical features, rendering the synthesized datasets sufficiently different from both the original and the image to be registered, they were included in cross-validation. With more subjects, the classification results may be further improved, and we could explore the popular convolutional neural networks to inspect the feature space and potentially improve the classification. Another limitation of the current techniques comes from the inter- and intra-variability of the scores in practice. With simple visual inspection of 3D data, it is challenging to establish consistent and accurate scores particularly for images that appear in between the categories (e.g., intermediate vs. good). This may partially contribute to the lower classification accuracy for the intermediate class, as many from the group were assigned to good/normal or poor groups. In addition, in contrast to the good/normal and poor collateral scores, the wider range of variability among the population of intermediate collateral circulation also contributes to the lower classification accuracy. However, in clinical practice, it is most important to differentiate between good and intermediate collaterals versus poor collateral circulation since in individuals with poor collaterals the results of thrombectomy are poor. In the future, we will conduct evaluation on the inter- and intra-rater variability in labelling collaterals, and further validate our technique in relation to such information. Although averaging the extracted blood vessels for each subject can help gain information regarding blood flow over time, we would like to explore other techniques that explore temporal information, as well as more advanced rank-reduction techniques that better preserve relevant features for more accurate collateral evaluation.

5   Conclusions

We have developed an automatic technique to compute a collateral circulation score with an overall 82.2% accuracy. To the best of our knowledge, this is the first time that a computer-assisted classification method has been used for this application, and it is the first step towards helping radiologists and neurosurgeons more efficiently and accurately determine the best course of treatment and predict patient outcomes.

References

1. Sharma, V.K., Teoh, H.L., Wong, L.Y., Su, J., Ong, B.K., Chan, B.P.: Recanalization therapies in acute ischemic stroke: pharmacological agents, devices, and combinations. Stroke Res. Treat. **2010** (2010)
2. Sung, S.M., Lee, T.H., Cho, H.J., Kang, T.H., Jung, D.S., Park, K.P., Park, M.K., Lee, J.I., Ko, J.K.: Functional outcome after recanalization for acute pure M1 occlusion of the middle cerebral artery as assessed by collateral CTA flow. Clin. Neurol. Neurosur. **131**, 72–76 (2015)
3. Ramaiah, S.S., Mitchell, P., Dowling, R., Yan, B.: Assessment of arterial collateralization and its relevance to intra-arterial therapy for acute ischemic stroke. J. Stroke Cerebrovasc. **23**, 399–407 (2014)
4. Cuccione, E., Padovano, G., Versace, A., Ferrarese, C., Beretta, S.: Cerebral collateral circulation in experimental ischemic stroke. Exp. Transl. Stroke Med. **8**, 2 (2016)
5. Pexman, J.H.W., Barber, P.A., Hill, M.D., Sevick, R.J., Demchuk, A.M., Hudon, M.E., Hu, W.Y., Buchan, A.M.: Use of the alberta stroke program early CT score (ASPECTS) for assessing CT scans in patients with acute stroke. Am. J. Neuroradiol. **22**, 1534–1542 (2001)
6. Fonov, V., Evans, A.C., Botteron, K., Almli, C.R., McKinstry, R.C., Collins, D.L., Brain Development Cooperative Group: Unbiased average age-appropriate atlases for pediatric studies. Neuroimage **54**, 313–327 (2011)
7. Cui, X., Huang, J., Zhang, S., Metaxas, Dimitris N.: Background subtraction using low rank and group sparsity constraints. In: Fitzgibbon, A., Lazebnik, S., Perona, P., Sato, Y., Schmid, C. (eds.) ECCV 2012. LNCS, vol. 7572, pp. 612–625. Springer, Heidelberg (2012). doi: 10.1007/978-3-642-33718-5_44

8. Lin, Z., Chen, M., Ma, Y.: The augmented Lagrange multiplier method for exact recovery of corrupted low-rank matrices. https://arxiv.org/abs/1009.5055
9. Turk, M., Pentland, A.: Eigenfaces for recognition. J. Cogn. Neurosci. **3**, 71–86 (1991)
10. Faruqe, M.O., Hasan, M.A.: Face recognition using PCA and SVM. In: Proceedings of the 3rd International Conference on Anti-Counterfeiting, Security, and Identification in Communication, pp. 97–101 (2009)

The Effect of Non-contrast CT Slice Thickness on Thrombus Density and Perviousness Assessment

M.L. Tolhuisen[1,2(✉)], J. Enthoven[1], E.M.M. Santos[1,2,3,4],
W.J. Niessen[3,4,5], L.F.M. Beenen[2], D.W.J. Dippel[6],
A. van der Lugt[3], W.H. van Zwam[7], Y.B.W.E.M. Roos[7],
R.J. van Oostenbrugge[8], C.B.L.M. Majoie[2], and H.A. Marquering[1,2]

[1] Biomedical Engineering and Physics, AMC, Amsterdam, The Netherlands
M.L.tolhuisen@amc.uva.nl
[2] Department of Radiology, AMC, Amsterdam, The Netherlands
[3] Department of Radiology, Erasmus MC, Rotterdam, The Netherlands
[4] Department of Medical Informatics, Erasmus MC, Rotterdam, The Netherlands
[5] Faculty of Applied Sciences, Delft, University of Technology, Delft, The Netherlands
[6] Department of Neurology, Erasmus MC, Rotterdam, The Netherlands
[7] Department of Radiology, Maastricht UMC, Maastricht, The Netherlands
[8] Department of Neurology, Maastricht UMC, Maastricht, The Netherlands
https://www.amc.nl/bmep

Abstract. [Background] It is expected that thrombus density and perviousness measurements are dependent on CT slice thickness, because density values are blurred in thicker slices. This study quantifies the effect of slice thickness on thrombus density and perviousness measurements. [Methods] Thrombus density and perviousness measurements were performed in 50 patients for varying slice thicknesses, using a manual and semi-automated technique. Linear regression was performed to determine the dependence of density measurements on slice thickness. Paired t-tests were used to test for differences in density and perviousness measures for varying slice thickness. [Results] Thrombus density decreased for increasing slice thickness with approximately 2HU per mm. Perviousness measurements were significantly higher for thick slice compared to thin slice NCCT. [Conclusion] Thick slice NCCT scans result in an underestimation of thrombus density and overestimation of thrombus perviousness.

Keywords: Ischemic stroke · Thrombus density · Thrombus perviousness · CT · Slice thickness

1 Introduction

Stroke has a major impact on society as it is one of the leading causes of death worldwide [1]. In 87% of all cases, stroke is caused by a thrombus that occludes an intracranial vessel (ischemic stroke) [2]. As a patient loses around 1.9 million neurons each minute, fast treatment to restore blood flow is crucial [3].

For the past years, research has focused on improving treatment for ischemic stroke. This resulted in endovascular treatment (EVT) as an addition to the standard treatment,

© Springer International Publishing AG 2017
M.J. Cardoso et al. (Eds.): CMMI/RAMBO/SWITCH 2017, LNCS 10555, pp. 168–175, 2017.
DOI: 10.1007/978-3-319-67564-0_17

after it showed increased functional outcome in several randomized clinical trials [4]. Nonetheless, patient outcome is still poor and further research is focusing on patient specific treatment selection, for example based on thrombus characteristics. It has been suggested that thrombus density measurements provide information on thrombus architecture and is a potential predictor for treatment effect [5]. In addition, Santos et al. [6, 7] showed that thrombus permeability was associated with higher recanalization rate and better functional outcome, after both EVT and IV-tPA.

Because the measurement permeability requires dynamic imaging, the definition thrombus perviousness was introduced as a measure to estimate thrombus permeability [6]. Perviousness is defined as the difference in thrombus voxel intensities, comparing CT angiography (CTA) to non-contrast CT (NCCT) [6]. In this assessment, imaging quality may be a limiting factor. Preferably, the assessment should be applied on low noise, high resolution, and thin slice images. In current clinical practice, thick slice NCCT images are commonly used because of lower noise levels and lower demand on storage capacity. CTA images have higher contrast to noise ratio and are therefor commonly stored as thin slices (approximately 1 mm thick). Because of averaging, which is applied to generate thick slice images, signal of small-scale structures such as thrombi may be reduced. Kim et al. [8] showed reduced sensitivity and specificity for thrombus detection on thick slice NCCT compared to thin slice NCCT. In this study we aim to quantify the effect of slice thickness on thrombus density and perviousness measurements.

2   Methods

2.1   Patient Selection

We included 50 consecutive patients from the Multicenter Randomize Clinical trial of Endovascular treatment of ischemic stroke in the Netherlands (MR CLEAN) cohort with thin slice ($\leq$2.5 mm) NCCT and CTA scans that were performed within 30 min on the same scanner.

2.2   Slice Reconstruction

Thick(er) slice images were reconstructed by taking the average over multiple thin slices for each voxel location. For a given slice thickness, multiple approaches can be followed to generate such an image. For example, if a new image is generated with twice as thick slice thickness, one can combine slice 1 and 2 or slice 2 and 3. Figure 1 illustrates how multiple approaches can be followed for thick slice reconstructions out of thin slices. First, all scans were super sampled to an initial slice thickness of 0.45 mm. Then, different reconstructions were created for given slice thicknesses. The resulted slice thicknesses ranged from 0.45 mm to 4.95 mm with an increment of 0.45 mm. The CTA slice thickness was kept at 0.45 mm.

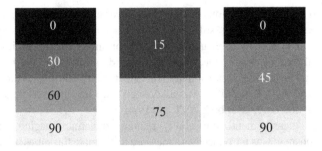

Fig. 1. Illustration of the slice reconstruction that is used to increase slice thickness. The numbers in the layers show examples of densities. This figures shows that to create a scan with a slice thickness twice as large as the original (Left), the example in the middle combined slice 1 and 2 and 3 and 4. The second example (Right) show the results when slice 2 and 3 are used to combined to generate an image with a thicker slice.

2.3   Density and Perviousness Measurements

Thrombus density measurements were initially performed on the original thin slice NCCT and CTA by a single expert observer, using both manual and semi-automated thrombus perviousness measurements described in [6, 9]. First, Elastix® [10] was used for rigid image registration to align the NCCT and CTA for each patient. For the manual density measurement, a spherical region of interest (ROI) with a radius of 1 mm was placed in the proximal, middle and distal part of the thrombus. The semi-automated perviousness measurements followed multiple steps. First, 2 ROIs were placed proximal and distal to the thrombus and symmetrically on the contralateral side. A coarse center-line of the contralateral vessel between the proximal and distal ROIs- was determined using a minimum cost path calculation on the CTA image filtered with a tuned Frangi's vesselness filter [11, 12]. Then, the vessel contour was obtained from this coarse center-line using a graph-cut segmentation technique with kernel regression [12]. The initial coarse centerline was corrected to be the center of mass of this segmented vessel contour and the radius along the fine centerline was determined. Finally, based on symmetry, the fine centerline was projected onto the occluded vessel using 3D-Bspline registration to optimize alignments. The same kernel regression segmentation technique was used on the CTA to segment the occluded vessel, guided by the aligned centerline. Due to a drop of intensity at the location of the thrombus, the radii of the segmented lumen decreases significantly. At the site of the thrombus, the vessel contours were replaced with the contralateral radius contours, thereby creating a shape prior. Within the shape prior, a combination of region growing segmentation and mathematical morphologies is used to obtain the final thrombus segmentation.

To assess thrombus perviousness, we used the thrombus attenuation increase (TAI), which is defined as the thrombus attenuation difference between CTA and NCCT measurements. The thrombus density measurements were obtained using the newly reconstructed NCCT images for all slice thicknesses. The density and perviousness measures for all slice thicknesses were compared to the original, thin slice, density and perviousness measurements.

2.4   Statistical Analysis

The mean and standard deviation of the difference in density measurements was calculated for each slice thickness. To investigate a potential correlation between thrombus density and slice thickness, a linear regression model was used based on the mean thrombus density for all patients. A paired t-test was used to investigate whether a significant difference in density and perviousness measurements was present, comparing the thin slice measurements to the measurements with the reconstructed scans with increased slice thicknesses.

All analyses were preformed using IBM® SPSS® Statistics software, version 24 (IBM Corp., Armonk, NY).

3   Results

Linear regression showed that the thrombus density values significantly decreased with increasing slice thickness. For each mm increase in slice thickness, the density measures decreased with 2.9 and 2.2 HU (both p < 0.001), for the manual measurements and the full thrombus segmentation respectively. Figure 2 shows the manual thrombus density measurements in 50 patients for varying slice thicknesses. The density measurements as assessed by the full thrombus segmentation are shown in Fig. 3.

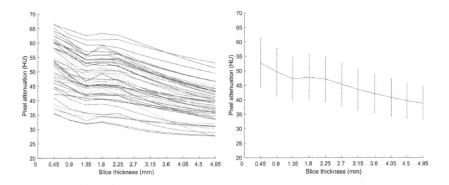

Fig. 2. (Left) NCCT thrombus density measures for varying slice thickness for 50 patients manually measured with ROIs; (Right) NCCT mean thrombus density for varying slice thickness measured with ROIs

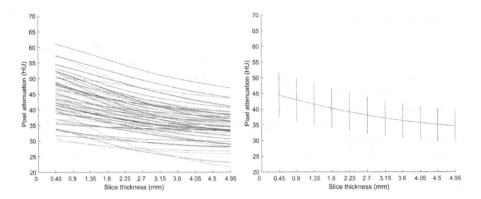

Fig. 3. (Left) NCCT thrombus density measures for varying slice thickness for 50 patients measured with the full thrombus segmentation; (Right) NCCT mean attenuation decrease over slice thickness measured with the full thrombus segmentation

The paired-t test showed that there was a significant decrease ($p < 0.001$) in thrombus perviousness measures for increasing slice thickness, comparing the thin-slice measurements with the measurement for NCCT with 0.9 mm slice thickness. Figures 4 and 5 show the results of the perviousness measurements in 50 patients for varying slice thicknesses, measured with the ROIs and full thrombus segmentation respectively.

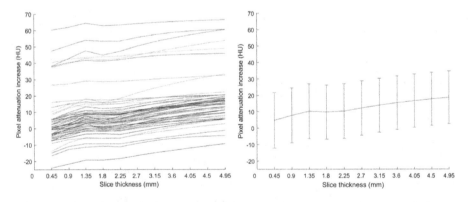

Fig. 4. (Left) Thrombus attenuation increase for varying slice thickness for 50 patients manually measured with ROIs; (Right) Mean attenuation increase over slice thickness measured with the ROIs

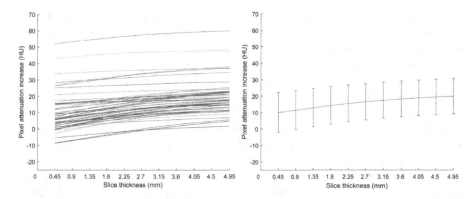

Fig. 5. (Left) Thrombus attenuation increase for varying slice thickness for 50 patients measured with the full thrombus segmentation; (Right) Mean attenuation increase over slice thickness measured with the full thrombus segmentation

4   Discussion

In this study, it was shown that there was a significant decrease in thrombus density measures with increasing CT slice thickness. As a result, perviousness measures increased with increasing NCCT slice thickness.

Thrombus characteristics, such as thrombus density and perviousness, may be used as treatment selection parameters or predictive parameters for treatment success and functional outcome for patients with ischemic stroke in the future [5–7]. While data storage will become a major challenge in the medical imaging field, it is important to know the consequences of data reduction [11]. This study showed that the increase of NCCT slice thickness resulted in reduced thrombus density and increased perviousness measurement values. Therefore, previous associations made between thrombus perviousness and favorable prognostics cannot be extrapolated for thick slice NCCT measurements, as they may lead to overestimation of favorable prognostics.

The results showed differences between the thrombus density and perviousness measurements, performed with the manual annotation compared to the semi-automated thrombus segmentation. Less variation was visible in the thrombus density and perviousness measurements between patients and the effect of increased slice thickness appeared less for the semi-automated full thrombus segmentation. This was expected because a larger volume of density values is included in this technique, which makes it less susceptible for noise.

The placement of ROIs in imaging data is easy applicable and can already be applied in daily clinical practice. However, it was shown that the full thrombus segmentation is less sensitive to slice thickness. Also, Santos et al. [12] showed a stronger association between thrombus perviousness and functional outcome and recanalization, based on full segmented thrombi measurements.

The linear regression showed an inverse relation between slice thickness and density measurements. This suggests that a correction for slice thickness could result in a more accurate density measurement.

A limitation of this study is that we did not correct for confounders. It could be possible that factors such as scanner manufacturer, reconstruction, size of thrombus, or filtering algorithms have influenced our results.

This study only used thrombus density and perviousness measurements from a single observer. Thereby, we did not take inter-observer variability into account. However, Santos et al. [9, 13] already showed reasonable inter-observer variability for both measurement techniques.

The increase of slice thickness creates a blurring effect in the z-direction. As a result, the decrease in density of the thrombus in the CT image is dependent on the orientation and fraction of the vessels present within the slice.

Longitudinal partial volume effect will be more apparent in thicker slices. Based on a phantom study, Monnin et al. [14] suggested that the optimal slice thickness is 75% of object width. As the average diameter of the M1 segment is 2.3 $\pm$ 0.3 mm and the vessel diameters are expected to decrease distally, this suggests a maximal slice thickness of approximately 1.7 mm [15]. However, we also see a reduction of thrombus densities with slice thickness between 0.45 and 1.7 mm.

5   Conclusion

This study showed that increasing NCCT slice thickness results in a decreasing thrombus density and an increase in thrombus perviousness assessment.

Acknowledgements. Part of this work has been founded by ITEA3 14003: Medolution.

References

1. Wang, H., Naghavi, M., Allen, C., Barber, R.M., Bhutta, Z.A.: Global, regional, and national life expectancy, all-cause mortality, and cause-specific mortality for 249 causes of death, 1980–2015: a systematic analysis for the Global Burden of Disease Study 2015. Lancet **388**(10053), 1459–1544 (2016)
2. American Heart Association, "Ischemic stoke" (2017). http://www.strokeassociation.org/STROKEORG/AboutStroke/TypesofStroke/IschemicClots/Ischemic-Strokes-Clots_UCM_310939_Article.jsp#.WSRFoevyhhE
3. Saver, J.L.: Time is brain-quantified. Stroke **37**(1), 263–266 (2006)
4. Goyal, M., et al.: Endovascular thrombectomy after large-vessel ischaemic stroke: A meta-analysis of individual patient data from five randomised trials. Lancet **387**(10029), 1723–1731 (2016)
5. Moftakhar, P., et al.: Density of thrombus on admission CT predicts revascularization efficacy in large vessel occlusion acute ischemic stroke. Stroke **44**, 243–246 (2013)
6. Santos, E.M.M., et al.: Thrombus permeability is associated with improved functional outcome and recanalization in patients with ischemic stroke. Stroke **47**(3), 732–741 (2016)

7. Santos, E.M.M., et al.: Permeable thrombi are associated with higher intravenous recombinant tissue-type plasminogen activator treatment success in patients with acute ischemic stroke. Stroke **47**(8), 2058–2065 (2016)
8. Eung, Y.K., et al.: Detection of thrombus in acute ischemic stroke: value of thin-section noncontrast-computed tomography. Stroke **36**(12), 2745–2747 (2005)
9. Santos, E.M.M., et al.: Development and validation of intracranial thrombus segmentation on CT angiography in patients with acute ischemic stroke. PLoS ONE **9**(7), 101985 (2014)
10. Klein, S., Staring, M., Murphy, K., Viergever, M.A., Pluim, J.P.W.: Elastix: a toolbox for intensity-based medical image registration. IEEE Trans. Med. Imaging **29**(1), 196–205 (2010)
11. Reinsel, D., Gantz, J., Rydning, J.: Data Age 2025: The Evolution of Data to Life-Critical Don't Focus on Big Data; Focus on the Data That's Big Sponsored by Seagate The Evolution of Data to Life-Critical Don't Focus on Big Data; Focus on the Data That's Big (2017)
12. Santos, E.M.M., Niessen, W.J., Yoo, A.J., Berkhemer, O.A.: Automated entire thrombus density measurements for robust and comprehensive thrombus characterization in patients with acute ischemic stroke. PLoS ONE **11**(1), 1–16 (2016)
13. Santos, E.M.M., et al.: Observer variability of absolute and relative thrombus density measurements in patients with acute ischemic stroke. Neuroradiology **58**(2), 133–139 (2016)
14. Monnin, P., Sfameni, N., Gianoli, A., Ding, S.: Optimal slice thickness for object detection with longitudinal partial volume effects in computed tomography. J. Appl. Clin. Med. Phys. **18**, 251–259 (2017)
15. Peter, R., Emmer, B.J., Van Es, A.C.G.M., Van Walsum, T.: Quantitative analysis of geometry and lateral symmetry of proximal middle cerebral artery. J. Stroke Cerebrovasc. Dis., 1–8 (2017)

Quantitative Collateral Grading on CT Angiography in Patients with Acute Ischemic Stroke

Anna M.M. Boers[1,2,3(✉)] ⓘ, Renan Sales Barros[1] ⓘ, Ivo G.H. Jansen[1,2] ⓘ,
Cornelis H. Slump[3] ⓘ, Diederik W.J. Dippel[4] ⓘ, Aad van der Lugt[5] ⓘ,
Wim H. van Zwam[6] ⓘ, Yvo B.W.E.M. Roos[8] ⓘ, Robert J. van Oostenbrugge[7] ⓘ,
Charles B.L.M. Majoie[2] ⓘ,
Henk A. Marquering[1,2] ⓘ, and on behalf of the MR CLEAN Investigators

[1] Department of Biomedical Engineering and Physics, AMC, Amsterdam, The Netherlands
a.m.m.boers@utwente.nl
[2] Department of Radiology and Nuclear medicine, AMC, Amsterdam, The Netherlands
[3] MIRA Institute for Biomedical Engineering and Technical Medicine, University of Twente, Enschede, The Netherlands
[4] Department of Neurology, Erasmus MC, Rotterdam, The Netherlands
[5] Department of Radiology, Erasmus MC, Rotterdam, The Netherlands
[6] Department of Radiology, Maastricht UMC, Maastricht, The Netherlands
[7] Departmentof Neurology, Maastricht UMC, Maastricht, The Netherlands
[8] Department of Neurology, AMC, Amsterdam, The Netherlands

Abstract. Reliable assessment of collateral blood supply is important in acute ischemic stroke. We propose a quantitative method for evaluation of collateral status on CT angiography (CTA). We collected CTA images of 70 patients from MR CLEAN with an occlusion in the M1 branch. Our proposed quantitative collateral score (qCS) consisted of atlas-based territory-at-risk identification and vessel segmentation using a Hessian-based filter. Ground truth was obtained by manual collateral scoring (mCS). Accuracy was evaluated by analysis of Spearman ρ and one-way ANOVA. Correlation of mCS and qCS with tissue death and functional outcome was assessed. Receiver operating characteristics curves of mCS and qCS were analyzed to distinguish favorable from unfavorable outcome. qCS strongly correlated with mCS and showed reliable correlations with tissue death and functional outcome. qCS showed higher discriminative power between favorable and unfavorable compared to mCS, indicating potential clinical value.

Keywords: Collateral status · Automatic assessment · Acute ischemic stroke · CT angiography · Endovascular therapy

1 Introduction

In stroke patients with acute proximal large vessel occlusion, endovascular therapy (EVT) and intravenous thrombolysis are the only two effective treatment options used in routine practice [1]. Many studies have emphasized the relevance of collateral assessment on baseline imaging to quickly identify patients who potentially benefit from EVT

© Springer International Publishing AG 2017
M.J. Cardoso et al. (Eds.): CMMI/RAMBO/SWITCH 2017, LNCS 10555, pp. 176–184, 2017.
DOI: 10.1007/978-3-319-67564-0_18

[2, 3]. Some studies even utilized the collateral status as an inclusion criteria for their randomized control trial [4]. Collaterals maintain blood flow via alternative routes in the brain and good collateral supply is associated with smaller infarct volumes and improved clinical outcome [5, 6]. To achieve information on the collateral status in the acute setting, single-phase CT angiography (CTA) is the most widely used imaging modality. Single-phase CTA is a snapshot of vascular contrast enhancement over time. Although information on dynamic filling of the leptomeningeal collaterals is lacking, CTA allows visualization of the extent of collateral capacity.

Many collateral grading systems on CTA have been proposed, but a consistent and easy to interpret standard score has yet to be found [7]. There is a need for objective and accurate collateral capacity assessment since current grading methods are susceptible to poor interobserver agreement and are often scored on coarse ordinal scales. An automated and quantitative collateral scoring method holds the promise to overcome these problems and aid in rapid triaging of patients for EVT. The aim of this study is to introduce a quantitative method for the evaluation of collateral status on CTA. We investigate the correlation of our proposed method with tissue and functional outcome and assess the predictive value for favorable functional outcome as compared to standard visual scoring.

2 Materials and Methods

2.1 Patient Selection

Study data was acquired from the MR CLEAN [8] database. Patient eligibility and methods of MR CLEAN have been described previously [9]. All patients or their legal representatives provided written informed consent. For this post-hoc analysis, we included 70 consecutive patients from the MR CLEAN database who received baseline thin-sliced single-phase CTA imaging (approximately 1 mm) and who had follow-up non-contrast CT (NCCT) imaging to allow follow-up infarct volume (FIV) assessment. No fixed CTA protocols were used in MR CLEAN, and protocols varied per center. We only included patients with an occlusion in the middle cerebral artery (MCA) M1 segment. Patients with large diffuse haemorrhagic transformations (PH2) and image data with extreme artifacts or insufficient scan quality were excluded. A summary of the clinical patient information is given in Table 1.

Table 1. Clinical baseline characteristics stratified by favorable and unfavorable outcome.

Parameter	All (N = 59)	mRS 0–2 (N = 22)	mRS 3–6 (N = 78)
Age (yr) (mean ± SD)	63.8 (13.5)	64.5 (15.1)	63.0 (13.5)
Sex (female) (No.,%)	24 (40.7)	6 (46.2)	18 (39.1)
NIHSS (median, IQR)	17 (14–21)	14 (9–17)	19 (16–22)
Onset to randomization (min) (median, IQR)	194 (145–282)	166 (132–233)	205 (148–291)

Note: NIHSS indicates National Institutes of Health Stroke Scale; IQR, interquartile range; mRS, modified Rankin Scale

2.2 Outcomes

The primary clinical outcome parameter was the patient's functional outcome at 90 days as captured by the mRS. The mRS is a 7-point scale ranging from no symptoms (score 0) to dead (score 6). Primary radiological outcome is the tissue outcome in terms of FIV assessed on follow-up NCCT. Secondary clinical outcome was the dichotomized mRS score of 0–2, which indicates functional independence and is considered a favorable outcome.

2.3 Manual Collateral Score

The presence of leptomeningeal collaterals on CTA was defined as relative differences in appearance of vasculature between hemispheres, distal to the proximal artery occlusion. In this study, the collateral status was scored manually on an existing commonly used ordinal scale by Tan et al. [10] as part of MR CLEAN and in a quantitative fashion using automatic analysis. In MR CLEAN, a central imaging committee assessed the manual collateral score (mCS) on baseline CTA. Image evaluators had more than 10 years of experience and were blinded to all clinical findings, except symptom side. All CTA images were independently graded by two neuroradiologists. A third reader resolved discrepancies between the initial two readers. The mCS was assessed on a commonly used 4-point scale, with 0 for absent collaterals (0% filling of the occluded territory), 1 for poor collaterals (>0% and $\leq$50% filling of the occluded territory), 2 for moderate (50% and <100% filling of the occluded territory), and 3 for good collaterals (100% filling of the occluded territory) [10]. Readers used the non-ischemic hemisphere as normal reference. A mixture of CTA images with NCCT window-level and maximum-intensity-projections were used for collateral grading, including all available slices. An example is shown in Fig. 1A. If different slices expressed different collateral capacities, an average collateral score over all slices was determined. No fixed CTA acquisition protocols were used in MR CLEAN and protocols varied per center. Inter-observer reliability for mCS assessment in MR CLEAN has previously been reported (kappa = 0.60) [5].

2.4 Quantitative Collateral Score

Quantitative collateral score (qCS) was obtained using an automatic method. This method uses CTA images as input and consisted of the following steps; (1) identification of affected territory at risk; (2) segmentation of vessels; and (3) comparison of vessel presence between hemispheres.

The location and extent of the territory at risk depends on the location of the intracranial occlusion. Inclusion of all vessels in the entire MCA territory might lead to overestimation of the collateral capacity. It is well-known that variation in cerebroarterial structures between patients is common, making precise territory at risk localization impossible without additional imaging. Therefore, the patient-specific territory at risk is estimated. Topographic probability maps as presented previously by Boers et al. [11] allow for identification of the area likely to infarct for a given occlusion location. These probability maps are created by the co-registration of individual follow-up NCCT images into the coordinate space of a healthy subject. FIVs per occlusion location were segmented, and mapped onto each other. The sum of the FIV masks represented the frequency of infarction for each voxel. Co-registration was performed to align the probability maps with each patient's CTA by a subsequent rigid and affine transformation. Mutual information was set as similarity measure. In this study, we focused on M1 occlusions and defined the territory at risk as the area that has >5% prevalence of infarction. This region is used as Region of Interest (ROI) and was mirrored to cover both the ipsilateral and contralateral side for further analysis (Fig. 1B).

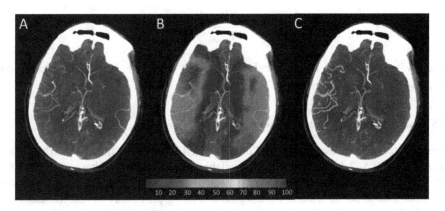

Fig. 1. **A**: Maximum intensity projection (MIP) of a CTA image with an occlusion in the left M1 branch and mCS of poor collaterals (>0% and ≤50% filling of the occluded territory). **B**: MIP with overlay of co-registered distribution map of infarct prevalence. Area of >5% is used as region of interest for the Hessian-based filter. **C**: MIP with segmented vessels distal to the M1 branch used for collateral capacity calculation. For this patient, the qCS was 27%.

After obtaining the ROIs in both hemispheres, a Hessian-based filter introduced by Frangi et al. [12] was applied to enhance tube-like structures (vessels) and suppress disk-like and blob-like structures. Because this filter is known for its sensitivity near edges, and thus the skull, a previously described skull-stripping algorithm was applied prior to filtering [13]. It is important to use a multi-scale approach to capture the variation in vessel size. For this, a detailed statistical cerebroarterial atlas that was derived from 700 normal MRA datasets [14] was used to obtain the mean vessel diameter distal to the M1 segment, ranging from 0.9 to 3.1 mm. This range was used as the input scale range for the filter. The step size for the multi-scale approach was set to 1.1 mm. The required parameters that control the sensitivity of the filter were chosen based on visual inspection and were set as $\alpha = 0.5$, $\beta = 0.5$, and $c = 500$. Filtering resulted in a 3D-image with a vesselness measure; each voxel in the output volume indicated the similarity of the local structure to a vessel. Applying a patient-specific threshold within the ROI on the vesselness image resulted in a binary image of the vessels. This threshold was defined as the mean + SD vesselness measure of the background; the area outside the ROI with a density of less than 200 Hounsfield units. A morphological closing operator using a disk-shaped structuring element with a radius of 0.4 mm was applied as post-processing step to correct for disconnected segments (Fig. 1C).

To ensure that only the vessels distal to the proximal M1 segment were measured, vessels with a diameter of >3.1 mm were excluded. Hereafter, the segmented vessels distal to the M1 segment in both hemispheres were extracted and multiplied by its density values (in Hounsfield units), where the sum represented the vascular presence (*VP*) of each hemisphere. The qCS was calculated as the percentage of the *VP* of the affected and healthy hemisphere via the following equation:

$$qCS = \max\left(100, \frac{VP_{ipsi}}{VP_{contra}}\right); 0 \le qCS \le 100$$

where VP_{ipsi} and VP_{contra} is the vascular presence of the affected and contralateral side respectively.

2.5   Assessment of Tissue Outcome

Tissue outcome was assessed on follow-up NCCT imaging, acquired 5–7 days after stroke onset. If 5–7 day NCCT was not available due to death or discharge, 24 h follow-up NCCT was used. In case of hemicraniectomy, the last scan prior to surgery was selected. The ischemic lesions were segmented using previously developed and validated software, resulting in a binary mask of the FIV [13]. Adjacent hyperdense areas suspected for hemorrhagic transformation were considered part of the FIV. All FIVs were inspected and adjusted if necessary by a trained observer (AMB) with more than 4 years of experience and at least one neuroradiologist (WvZ, LFB or CBM) with more than 15 years of experience. A consensus reading with 2 neuroradiologists was performed to resolve cases with any discrepancies. FIV was calculated in milliliters (mL) by multiplying the number of voxels of the segmented ischemic lesions with its voxel size.

Table 2. Tissue outcome and collateral scores

Variable	All (N = 59)	mRS 0–2 (N = 22)	mRS 3–6 (N = 78)
FIV (median, IQR)	88 (31–215)	23 (9–30)	116 (34–249)
mCS (mean ± SD)	1.8 (1.0)	2.5 (0.8)	1.6 (0.9)
qCS (mean ± SD)	47.9 (31.9)	40.6 (30.9)	73.3 (21.2)

Note:– FIV indicates follow-up infarct volume; mCS, manual collateral score; qCS, quantitative collateral score; mRS, modified Rankin Scale

2.6   Statistical Analysis

Dichotomous variables were presented as proportion of population. Continuous variables were tested for normality (Kolmogorov–Smirnov test) and presented as mean and SD if normally distributed or as median and interquartile range (IQR) otherwise. The mCS was used as a reference standard to evaluate the accuracy of the proposed qCS method. The accuracy was assessed by constructing boxplots and calculation of the Spearman rank correlation coefficients. One-way ANOVA analysis was performed to test for differences in qCS between mCS groups.

Receiver operating characteristics (ROC) curves were created and the area under the curve (AUC) was calculated to quantify the discriminative power of mCS and qCS to distinguish between favorable and unfavorable functional outcome (mRS 0–2 versus mRS 3–6). Sensitivity and specificity were calculated. All statistical analyses were performed in SPSS v.24.0 (IBM Corp., Armonk, NY, USA). A p-value of <0.05 indicated statistical significance in all analyses.

3 Results

We included 70 patients with an M1 occlusion in the MCA territory. We additionally excluded 11 patients due to incomplete head scans (n = 7), extreme movement artifacts (n = 2) and errors in co-registration (n = 2), resulting in a total of 59 patients for analysis. Mean age was 63.8 (SD ± 13.4), mean slice thickness was 0.89 mm (SD ± 0.17), and median FIV was 81 mL (IQR:31-214.5).

The correlation between qCS and mCS was significant with a Spearman ρ of 0.68, p < 0.001. Boxplots are displayed per mCS grade in Fig. 2. The qCS was significantly different between all mCS groups, except for absent collaterals (grade 0) versus poor collaterals (grade 1). Imaging parameters are shown in Table 2.

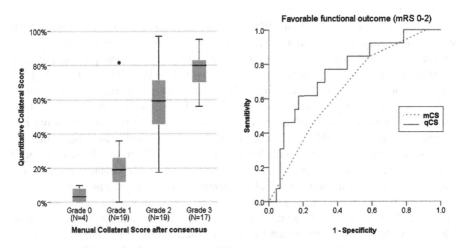

Fig. 2. Left: distribution of quantitative collateral score (qCS) per manual collateral score (mCS) grade, ranging from absent collaterals (0% filling of the occluded territory) to good collaterals (100% filling of the occluded territory). The qCS was significantly different between all mCS groups, except for absent collaterals (grade 0) versus poor collaterals (grade 1). Right: ROC curve analysis of mCS and qCS for discriminating favorable outcome (mRS 0–2) from unfavorable outcome (mRS 3–6).

The correlation of qCS and mCS with FIV were similar (both Spearman $\rho = -0.61$, $p < 0.001$). Correlation with mRS as outcome measure was also significant for both collateral scores; qCS showed Spearman $\rho = 0.36$, $p = 0.006$; and mCS showed Spearman $\rho = 0.28$, $p = 0.03$. ROC curves are displayed in Fig. 2. The discriminative power of mCS to distinguish between favorable and unfavorable functional outcome was poor with an AUC of 0.66. The proposed qCS showed an AUC of 0.76, representing a fair discriminative power, with a sensitivity and specificity of respectively 0.77 and 0.67.

4   Discussion

We have presented a new quantitative method to estimate the collateral capacity on CTA imaging of patients with an acute ischemic stroke. We have shown that the quantitative score strongly correlates with the manual collateral score. In our population, the associations of the quantitative collateral score with clinical and radiological outcome is identical to the common manual score, indicating the great potential clinical value.

To our knowledge, this is the first study that quantifies collateral capacity on CTA imaging. Visualization of the collateral capacity is not limited to CTA, and grading methods on various imaging modalities have been introduced. Four-vessel Digital subtraction angiography (DSA) is considered the gold standard for assessment of collateral supply. However, in the process of rapidly triaging patients for stroke therapy, DSA is seldom used because of its invasiveness and time-consuming nature [3, 15, 16]. Ernst and colleagues [17] previously introduced an atlas-based method for TOF- and contrast-enhanced MRA imaging to score collateral abundance in a quantitative fashion. Despite promising results, it might be challenging to translate these results to other types of imaging protocols.

Our study has some limitations. We only selected patients with a proven M1 occlusion for this study, resulting in a selection bias. Though the M1 segment of the MCA territory is the most common location for a large vessel occlusion, our proposed method should prove accurate for other occlusion types as well to be utilized in the total EVT eligible population. Furthermore, this study suffers from a relative small number of subjects which impedes multivariable regression analysis. Important prognostic factors, such as age, baseline National Institutes of Health Stroke Scale (NIHSS) score and treatment allocation should be included in future studies to further investigate the role of qCS assessment in acute stroke. We used thin-slice CTA to proof our concept of quantitative collateral scoring and applying our method on CTA images with thicker slices might result in suboptimal vessel segmentation, impairing the final qCS.

Our method heavily depends on the output of the Hessian-based filter introduced by Frangi et al. [12], the so-called vesselness filter. It is known that traditional Hessian-based filters often fail in preserving the vessel structure during smoothing, and small vessels and bifurcations might be characterized as background. Despite these disadvantages, we chose to use Frangi's vesselness filter for several reasons: (1) it was designed to detect vessels in angiography images; (2) it addresses the multiscale character of artery trees, thereby accounting for variations in vessel diameters; and (3) small flaws in detecting vascular structures would only result in minimal loss of accuracy, since our approach compares hemispheres to obtain the final qCS. In this study, we did not compare other Hessian-based filters or other filter types such as linear and non-linear anisotropic filters. Furthermore, the optimal sensitivity parameters for the vesselness filter were set according to visual inspection. Exploring the output of different setting and filters might result in an even more robust and accurate method, and will be addressed in a future study.

In this study, a quantitative method to estimate the collateral capacity in automated fashion on CTA is presented. There is a strong correlation with the manual reference score and our method showed strong correlations with tissue death and functional outcome. Quantitative scoring showed higher discriminative power between favorable and unfavorable outcome after stroke in comparison to manual assessment, and might be helpful in future patient selection models for EVT.

Funding. Anna MM Boers and Ivo GH Jansen are supported by a grant from the Stichting Toegepast Wetenschappelijk Instituut voor Neuromodulatie (TWIN). The MR CLEAN trial was funded by the Dutch Heart Foundation and through unrestricted grants from AngioCare BV, Covidien/EV3, MEDAC Gmbh/LAMEPRO and Penumbra Inc.

References

1. Goyal, M., Menon, B.K., van Zwam, W.H., et al.: Endovascular thrombectomy after large-vessel ischaemic stroke: a meta-analysis of individual patient data from five randomised trials. Lancet (London, England) (2016). doi:10.1016/S0140-6736(16)00163-X
2. Menon, B.K., Smith, E.E., Modi, J., et al.: Regional leptomeningeal score on ct angiography predicts clinical and imaging outcomes in patients with acute anterior circulation occlusions. Am. J. Neuroradiol. **32**, 1640–1645 (2011). doi:10.3174/ajnr.A2564
3. Christoforidis, G.A., Mohammad, Y., Kehagias, D., et al.: Angiographic assessment of pial collaterals as a prognostic indicator following intra-arterial thrombolysis for acute ischemic stroke. AJNR Am. J. Neuroradiol. **26**, 1789–1797 (2005)
4. Goyal, M., Demchuk, A.M., Menon, B.K., et al.: Randomized assessment of rapid endovascular treatment of ischemic stroke. N. Engl. J. Med. **372**, 1019–1030 (2015). doi: 10.1056/NEJMoa1414905
5. Berkhemer, O.A., Jansen, I.G.H., Beumer, D., et al.: Collateral status on baseline computed tomographic angiography and intra-arterial treatment effect in patients with proximal anterior circulation stroke. Stroke **47**, 768–776 (2016). doi:10.1161/STROKEAHA.115.011788
6. Boers, A.M., Jansen, I.G., Berkhemer, O.A., et al.: Collateral status and tissue outcome after intra-arterial therapy for patients with acute ischemic stroke. J. Cereb. Blood Flow Metab. (2016). doi:10.1177/0271678X16678874
7. McVerry, F., Liebeskind, D.S., Muir, K.W.: Systematic review of methods for assessing leptomeningeal collateral flow. Am. J. Neuroradiol. **33**, 576–582 (2012). doi:10.3174/ajnr.A2794
8. Berkhemer, O., Fransen, P., Beumer, D., et al.: A randomized trial of intraarterial treatment for acute ischemic stroke. New Engl. J. Med. **372**, 11–20 (2015). doi:10.1056/NEJMoa1411587

9. Fransen, P.S., Beumer, D., Berkhemer, O.A., et al.: MR CLEAN, a multicenter randomized clinical trial of endovascular treatment for acute ischemic stroke in the Netherlands: study protocol for a randomized controlled trial. Trials **15**, 343 (2014). doi:10.1186/1745-6215-15-343

10. Tan, I.Y.L., Demchuk, A.M., Hopyan, J., et al.: CT angiography clot burden score and collateral score: correlation with clinical and radiologic outcomes in acute middle cerebral artery infarct. Am. J. Neuroradiol. **30**, 525–531 (2009). doi:10.3174/ajnr.A1408

11. Boers, A.M.M., Berkhemer, O.A., Slump, C.H., et al.: Topographic distribution of cerebral infarct probability in patients with acute ischemic stroke: mapping of intra-arterial treatment effect. J. Neurointerv. Surg. (2016). doi:10.1136/neurintsurg-2016-012387

12. Frangi, A.F., Niessen, W.J., Vincken, K.L., Viergever, M.A.: Multiscale Vessel Enhancement Filtering, pp. 130–137. Springer, Heidelberg (1998)

13. Boers, A.M., Marquering, H.A., Jochem, J.J., et al.: Automated cerebral infarct volume measurement in follow-up noncontrast CT scans of patients with acute ischemic stroke. AJNR Am. J. Neuroradiol. **34**, 1522–1527 (2013). doi:10.3174/ajnr.A3463

14. Forkert, N.D., Fiehler, J., Suniaga, S., et al.: A statistical cerebroarterial atlas derived from 700 MRA datasets. Methods Inf. Med. **52**, 467–474 (2013). doi:10.3414/ME13-02-0001

15. Jansen, I.G.H., Berkhemer, O.A., Yoo, A.J., et al.: Comparison of CTA- and DSA-based collateral flow assessment in patients with anterior circulation stroke. Am. J. Neuroradiol. **37**(11), 2037–2042 (2016)

16. Elijovich, L., Goyal, N., Mainali, S., et al.: CTA collateral score predicts infarct volume and clinical outcome after endovascular therapy for acute ischemic stroke: a retrospective chart review. J. Neurointerv. Surg. **8**, 1–4 (2015)

17. Ernst, M., Forkert, N.D., Brehmer, L., et al.: Prediction of infarction and reperfusion in stroke by flow- and volume-weighted collateral signal in MR angiography. AJNR Am. J. Neuroradiol. **36**, 275–282 (2015). doi:10.3174/ajnr.A4145

Author Index

Printed in the United States
By Bookmasters